WHY
BIRTH TRAUMA
MATTERS

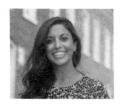

About the author

Dr Emma Svanberg has worked as a psychologist for 10 years, specialising in work with parents and parents-to-be during pregnancy, birth and the early years. During this work, she realised that many clients were seeking her help because they had experienced a difficult start to their parenting journey, or related to their previous experiences of trauma. This led to a particular interest in the transition to parenthood and the experience of birth, and Emma started blogging and using social media to spread awareness of the frequency of these experiences – with the hope of letting parents know that they are not alone.

In 2017 Emma ran a campaign on social media called #makebirthbetter, gathering women's experiences of birth. This brought her into contact with Dr Rebecca Moore, and together they founded Make Birth Better, an organisation devoted to reducing the impact of birth trauma.

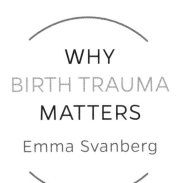

WHY
BIRTH TRAUMA
MATTERS

Emma Svanberg

pinter
&
martin

Why Birth Trauma Matters (Pinter & Martin Why It Matters 15)

First published by Pinter & Martin Ltd 2019
Reprinted 2021

ISBN 978-1-78066-610-5

Also available as an ebook

Pinter & Martin Why It Matters ISSN 2056-8657
Series editor: Susan Last
Index: Helen Bilton
Author photograph: Phill Taylor

British Library Cataloguing-in-Publication Data

A catalogue record for this book is available from the British Library.

Set in Minion

Printed and bound in the EU by Hussar

This book has been printed on paper that is sourced and harvested from sustainable forests and is FSC accredited.

Pinter & Martin Ltd
6 Effra Parade
London SW2 1PS

pinterandmartin.com

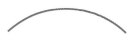

Contents

Acknowledgements	6
Author's Note	7
Introduction: It's Not Just About a Healthy Baby	9
1 What is Trauma?	15
2 Birth Trauma: A Silent Epidemic	23
3 Experiencing Birth Trauma	46
4 The Second Victim	65
5 Healing	86
6 The Next Baby	124
7 Changing the Culture of Birth	138
Seeking Help	143
References	145
Index	153

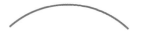

Acknowledgements

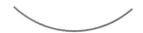

There are far too many people to thank. All of the women and birthing people I have met during my career so far and their partners, babies and families who have all taught me what birth trauma is. The 75 women who shared their stories with me and taught me how wide-reaching the impact of birth trauma can be. And all of the parents and professionals who contribute to Make Birth Better and have helped me think about how preventable birth trauma is and how much support can help.

Particular thanks to Becca, Caroline, Nikki and Jan for everything you do to make birth better.

Thanks to the Svanbergs and the Jankels.

And thanks to my square family for being my biggest teachers.

Author's Note

Many of the themes and stories in this book are difficult to read. If you are struggling, please put this book down and talk to someone. This might be a friend or family member, or you might want to make an appointment to see a healthcare professional or therapist.

Please read with care, being mindful of your response. If you need to take a break, please do.

Throughout the book I have tried to use the terminology 'women and birthing people' to acknowledge transgender and non-gender-conforming people who give birth. At the time of writing, there is very little research into the experiences of transgender and non-gender-conforming people, which is reflected in the content of the book.

'I think your first birth delivers you into motherhood. It is literally the gateway to your mother self. I can pretty much spot the mothers who have had a hard time and those that have had a positive experience. One feels empowered, the other feels bereft.'

Jenna – Mum, doula, Make Birth Better contributor

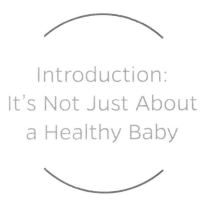

Introduction:
It's Not Just About
a Healthy Baby

Birth. It's just one day in your life. Or maybe sometimes four days, but really it's just a means to an end, isn't it? You should do whatever you're told, and go with the flow, don't expect too much so you won't be disappointed. But don't expect any support from midwives or doctors, because they're too busy. All those natural birth stories are just for hippies: birth is meant to be painful. But if you don't think positively then you'll be anxious, and that will harm your baby and lead to a difficult birth. Anyway, regardless of your experience, as long as the baby ends up OK you should be happy. What have you got to complain about?

When you look at how we talk about birth in modern UK society, it seems almost inevitable that people begin their journey to birth feeling confused, unsupported and afraid. There are a number of conflicting messages. The first is that women are vessels for their babies, so should not consider their own needs during the expulsion of that baby from their body. The second is that women are goddesses, and should expect nothing less than an empowering experience from their birth. A third is that birth is inherently safe and can be done alone at home by following your instincts. A fourth is that birth is inherently risky and must be done on a labour ward with doctors nearby. A fifth is that birth is a painful ordeal that must be managed and got through. Yet another is that birth is orgasmic and joyful. And all of this is happening in the context of services that are, on the one hand, going through a major transformation, and, on the other, suffering from a severe lack of resources. Is it any wonder, then, that people are increasingly coming out of their birth experience feeling shaken and shocked? And because of yet another message – that as long as we all survived, we should be happy – they feel unable to talk about that shock.

But birth does matter. It is the door to our journey to parenthood. How we feel about our birth colours our entire parenting experience. Do we start off feeling empowered or broken? We are increasingly talking about maternal mental health problems, and more funding is going into secondary care perinatal services than ever before. But so many of these problems are underpinned by difficult experiences during birth. If we can improve birth we can prevent problems developing, not only for those giving birth, but also for their partners and children.

When I first began seeing parents for individual talking therapy, one of the biggest surprises was how many of them had been through difficult birth experiences. At that time not a mother myself, I sat through countless stories of women birthing alone on a labour ward with no midwife available, women haemorrhaging unexpectedly and having flashbacks and nightmares about drowning in blood, families continuing to live with the impact of birth injuries sustained years before, and couples treated with contempt by those they had expected to care for them. Many people, at some time during their birth, had felt certain they or their babies would not come out the other side. Their partners too had been left horrified by what they had witnessed and the helplessness they had experienced. During my psychological training, no one had ever mentioned the influence of birth on a parent's mental health. But once I started asking, supporting parents in recovering from a difficult birth experience became central to much of my therapeutic work.

Fast forward 10 years and, on the surface, things have changed. Around the country, there are huge changes to Maternity Services as part of the Maternity Transformation Programme, with an emphasis on continuity and personalisation of care. The recent WHO recommendations, on intrapartum care for a positive childbirth experience, place the woman or birthing person, and the baby, firmly at the centre. The Improving Access to Psychological Therapies programme, a national programme to provide easy access to talking therapies, is developing a specialist perinatal workforce to support parents and parents-to-be in a primary care setting (within GP surgeries, Children's Centres and local organisations). And there has been an enormous increase in funding for perinatal mental health services as part of the NHS Five Year Forward Plan, which will be expanded as part of the NHS long-term plan. All of this is designed to support parents at risk of mental health difficulties during the perinatal period (during pregnancy, and in the first year of parenthood), including those who feel traumatised by their birth or are at risk of finding birth traumatic.

However, many still feel that support is not there, or when it is, it is hard to find. While funding is being injected into secondary care services such as Mother and Baby Units, this is not yet nationwide and many people who do not meet the criteria for these services fall through the gaps. Parents referred to primary care services may be told they aren't eligible for therapy, or face a long wait (sometimes longer than the pregnancy they are requesting help with), or be seen by a practitioner without specialist perinatal training or supervision. In some areas, people can access Specialist Mental Health Midwives. In others, midwives have little mental health training and feel ill equipped to manage such difficulties. And when people *are* offered support for recovering from a birth trauma, this may be within the team of midwives or even in the hospital in which they were traumatised. When parents do access help, it may be with a practitioner who is burnt out and disillusioned. Support for birth partners is rarely available. And too often, when people are brave enough to reach out and talk about their experience, the response is that same old 'Well, you should be happy you have a healthy baby', adding to the shame of the experience and making it even less likely they will seek support again.

Further, as well as thinking about how to *support* families with mental health difficulties after birth (and families whose mental health difficulties have been *caused* by birth), we also need to think about how to *prevent* mental health difficulties. As users of maternity services, we need to be aware of what we are entitled to, the choices we have, and the factors that can influence our birth outcomes. As individuals, we are at a critical time when we can influence local and national policy and get involved in creating radical change. And as a society, we can start to discuss birth openly and honestly, inviting people to share their experiences to encourage not just learning, but healing too.

And why does it matter that we talk about birth? While statistics suggest that at least 1–4% of women experience PTSD (Post-Traumatic Stress Disorder) after birth, we know that many more suffer from traumatic symptoms and up to 60% of women experience a 'negative birth experience'.

What statistics don't demonstrate is how far-reaching the effects of a difficult birth can be. If birth is the door to parenthood, a positive experience can fill us with confidence in our body, leaving us feeling powerful and proud, prepared to face new challenges. A difficult or traumatic experience can knock us completely, affecting our relationships, our trust in services, our sense of self and our physical health. With a new baby to look after, and no time to process the experience, it can stay with us for years.

This book will explore what birth trauma is, and how it can affect people. It will consider how far-reaching trauma can be, affecting not only mothers and their partners, but also their babies, members of staff in maternity services and wider society. I'll talk about how you can begin to heal from a difficult birth experience – the different therapeutic options available to you, as well as support groups and charities – and how to make a complaint if you feel you've been let down by services. This book is aimed at women, birthing people and their partners who have had a difficult experience. If you would like to read about how to increase your chances of a positive birth, take a look at *The Positive Birth Book* by Milli Hill and *How to Have a Baby* by Natalie Meddings. I have focused mainly on women in writing this book, because proportionally they are most affected by difficult births. But hearing the voices of partners who have witnessed a traumatic birth is also crucial. If you would like to read more about this, please take a look at the work of Dr Andy Mayers. So far, very little has been written about the experiences of transgender and non-gender-conforming people in their birth and postnatal journey, although what has been written suggests that the increased stigma they face could increase their risk of experiencing birth and the maternity system as traumatic.

My hope is that this book will be part of a new approach not only to birth trauma, but to birth itself. By acknowledging how important birth is, and what happens when it goes wrong, we can start to see how easily trauma could be prevented. Too often, a kind word or a loving touch would have made all the difference. It wouldn't take much to ensure that parents embark on their journey feeling pride instead of shame.

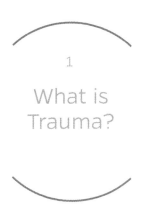

1

What is Trauma?

Before we begin talking about birth trauma, it's important that we understand what is meant by the word 'trauma'. It's a word that gets heard more frequently these days, with a rise in awareness of Post-Traumatic Stress Disorder (PTSD) following the wars in Iraq and Afghanistan; greater discussion of traumatic stress symptoms following incidents such as the Grenfell fire, the London bombings and the World Trade Center; the recognition that many problems – both psychological and physical – throughout a person's life may be due to Adverse Childhood Experiences (ACEs), and even social media warning us of possible 'triggers' in published posts. Perhaps there is a greater awareness that experiences that leave us feeling fundamentally unsafe have long-lasting repercussions. People even joke about trauma – saying they feel 'traumatised' by a bad haircut or the final of *Love Island*.

But what is 'trauma', really, and how can it affect us?

What is trauma?

Trauma as a concept has only been around since 1980, with the inclusion of Post-Traumatic Stress Disorder (PTSD) as a diagnosis in the *Diagnostic and Statistical Manual of Mental Disorders* (DSM-III), the manual used worldwide to diagnose mental health problems. Until 1980, it was thought that psychological disorders were caused by something within our character or biology, rather than by an external event.

The definition of trauma has been remarkably controversial (Brewin et al, 2009), with some psychologists suggesting that, because trauma is so varied and subjective, it might be better not to define it at all, but instead look purely at the symptoms it can cause. Using the DSM, we see trauma as being caused by a particular difficult event – or a 'stressor'. We have learned since 1980 that our reactions to this stressor can vary widely, and differ depending on our individual vulnerabilities; the things that make us uniquely susceptible, such as a previous history of other traumatic events. We also know now that we can respond to a traumatic event which we haven't experienced ourselves, such as by witnessing an event or through hearing about it. And sometimes a traumatic reaction isn't just caused by one particular event, but by a prolonged stressful situation (such as harassment at work).

The most recent version of the DSM, the fifth edition (DSM-V, 2013) defines a 'traumatic stressor' as follows:

'The person was exposed to: death, threatened death, actual or threatened serious injury, or actual or threatened sexual violence, in the following way(s):
- *Direct exposure*
- *Witnessing the trauma*
- *Learning that a relative or close friend was exposed to a trauma*

- *Indirect exposure to aversive details of the trauma, usually in the course of professional duties (e.g., first responders, medics)'*

It is generally accepted that this might include a perceived threat to yourself or someone else. What is key is the *threat to our sense of safety.*

The most recent version of the *International Classification of Diseases* (ICD-11), published by the World Health Organization to outline all health conditions (not just psychiatric ones) has a broader definition of a stressor: *'extremely threatening or horrific event or series of events'.* From bullying at work to living in a war zone, what defines trauma is how we respond to it. Trauma therefore becomes an entirely subjective concept, only able to be defined by those who have experienced it.

'Achieving a consensus definition of trauma is essential for progress in the field of traumatic stress. However, creating an all-purpose, general definition has proven remarkably difficult. Stressors vary along a number of dimensions, including magnitude (which itself varies on a number of dimensions, e.g., life threat, threat of harm, interpersonal loss; cf. Green, 1993), complexity, frequency, duration, predictability, and controllability. At the extremes, i.e., catastrophes versus minor hassles, different stressors may seem discrete and qualitatively distinct, but there is a continuum of stressor severity and there are no crisp boundaries demarcating ordinary stressors from traumatic stressors. Further, perception of an event as stressful depends on subjective appraisal, making it difficult to define stressors objectively, and independent of personal meaning making.' Weathers & Keane, 2007

When does trauma turn to traumatised?

Studying trauma, as you can imagine, can leave you with a

slightly skewed view of the world. You end up reading a lot about horrific events such as sexual abuse, war, terrorism and disaster. But there is a lot of hope too, in the growing research that looks at what makes us resilient in the face of trauma, and how we can continue to grow and develop despite experiencing traumatic events. While 50–60% of people throughout Europe experience a traumatic event at some point in their lifetime, only about 10% go on to develop PTSD (Horn et al., 2016; in Ayers, 2017).

Many people will have an *acute stress reaction* to a traumatic event, which might share many of the similar features of PTSD such as feeling very anxious, having trouble sleeping, or wanting to withdraw socially. The difference is that, for most people, these symptoms will gradually disappear once the person feels safe again. If they continue for more than a month after the event has passed, we might begin to say that someone is traumatised; that they are suffering from PTSD.

PTSD is what happens when we experience a cluster of different symptoms which last for at least a month. According to the DSM-V there are four different criteria related to symptoms, and to be diagnosed with PTSD you will be experiencing at least one symptom in each category – and will have experienced them for at least a month and to the extent that they are interfering with normal life. Criterion A is the traumatic stressor, and the other criteria are as follows:

Criterion B – Re-experiencing
You will have at least one symptom where you feel that you are frequently going over the event. These may include unwanted, upsetting memories, nightmares, flashbacks or feeling upset at reminders of the event. Some researchers say that this is the defining feature of PTSD, and what makes it stand apart from other disorders. It's also one of the key symptoms focused on in therapies for trauma.

Criterion C – Avoidance
You will have at least one symptom concerned with trying to avoid anything to do with the event. This may mean avoiding talking about the event, or even allowing yourself to think about it. You might also avoid anything which reminds you of the trauma.

Criterion D – Negative thoughts or feelings
You will have at least two symptoms related to the way you think about the stressor. This covers a wide range of experiences, related to your memories of the event (you may find it hard to remember parts of it), your appraisals (blaming yourself or other people for causing it to happen), or more general symptoms such as feeling low in mood.

Criterion E – Arousal and reactivity
Again, you would have at least two symptoms related to your responses to situations, such as feeling unusually irritable, having difficulty sleeping and feeling very alert to threat.

It is worth knowing that there has been a dramatic change in the criteria used to assess PTSD between DSM-IV and V, with the removal of Criterion A2. The main change has been that, prior to 2013, to be diagnosed with PTSD you needed to have experienced a traumatic event that involved 'actual or threatened death or serious injury, or a threat to the physical integrity of self or others' (criterion A1) *and* also responded to this with intense fear, helplessness, or horror (criterion A2). This change may have increased the number of people who would now meet the criteria for PTSD.

So why do some people recover from trauma, while others can be affected for years after the event?

How we understand trauma

There are two main models for understanding trauma and PTSD, which go some way to explaining why some people continue to suffer and others recover quickly.

The first concerns why PTSD symptoms occur, and relates to how we process trauma at the time of the event. This is called the 'dual representation theory' and Chris Brewin, Professor of Clinical Psychology at UCL, has elaborated on it over the last 20 years to encompass newer knowledge about how the brain processes trauma. When we experience normal events, they are processed using our episodic memory (literally, categorising events into different episodes such as 'times we went to the beach' and 'times we felt loved'). These utilise a part of the brain called the hippocampus, and can be easily accessed later on.

In contrast, when we experience a traumatic event the hippocampus goes pretty much offline and the amygdala comes into play. This is the alarm system in our brains, which kicks in our sympathetic nervous system and gets us out of danger quickly. It raises our cortisol (stress hormone) levels, raises our heart rate and sends blood rushing to our limbs so we can either fight, run away or freeze. This is survival mode, and in order to work effectively it also switches off the more sophisticated parts of our brain. Because our attention is focused entirely on the danger, the other things in our environment aren't tied together in our memories, making them very fragmented (this explains the changes we experience in our thoughts and memories later on). And because they've been stored by the amygdala, and not neatly filed away by the hippocampus, they're not easy to access. One of the areas which switches off during a traumatic experience is Broca's area, involved in language – meaning we can't put our experience into words.

Instead, the memories come bursting out when we're

reminded of them, or in nightmares. This is why you might find it really hard to remember details of an event until you walk into the room in which it happened, at which point it feels like it's happening all over again. For some, the experience feels so horrific they essentially go offline completely, which we call dissociation. This protects us at the time of the event, but means memories can feel even more fragmented.

Pierre Janet described it perfectly when he said:

'memories of traumatic experiences are dissociated or split off from normal consciousness, resulting in powerful and uncontrollable re-enactments.' (in Brewin, 2015)

The second main model, by Anke Ehlers and David Clark (2000), focuses more on the attribution we give to the traumatic event, and why it may then continue to affect us. While Brewin's theory considers memory, this model looks at meaning.

Ehlers and Clark suggest that traumatic symptoms become long lasting because the stressor is processed in a way that makes us feel that we – or those around us – are still in danger. This is due in part to the way the memory has been stored, but also how we have made sense of the event and how we continue to deal with it. Trauma is more likely to affect us long term if, at the time, it affects the way we see ourselves and the world rather than as a one-off unusual situation. For example, 'this world is a dangerous place' or 'I attract danger'. This means we continue to feel threatened even when we are objectively safe. We then use strategies, such as isolating ourselves from other people, or pushing away traumatic memories because they feel too disturbing, to protect ourselves. However, these strategies have the unwanted effect of maintaining the PTSD because we can never challenge the meaning we are making.

This model has been instrumental in the development of treatments for PTSD, and is the basis of Cognitive Behavioural

Therapy (CBT) for PTSD, which I will describe further in Chapter 5.

We know that some people are more likely to develop PTSD than others, due to their own individual circumstances (which in Ehlers and Clark's model would be the cause of negative appraisals). People who have had previous experiences of trauma, such as those who have experienced abuse or neglect in their childhoods, are at increased risk of developing PTSD following another traumatic event. Factors around the event matter too – if you go into a state of helplessness or dissociate you're also more likely to develop PTSD. And those who have little social support around them, understandably, are more likely to develop PTSD (one way of explaining this might be that there is no one to challenge the negative appraisals that have been made).

The ICD-11 also defines 'complex PTSD', which leads to fundamental personal changes: the way we relate to ourselves, our emotions and our relationships, usually due to repeated or chronic traumatic events (such as childhood abuse). In contrast, others may have some but not all of the criteria symptoms of PTSD, meaning that they live without a diagnosis but struggle to manage with such difficult symptoms.

We can think of trauma as something that can switch on our survival mode, and in some people this doesn't get switched off again. If you want to read more about it, Bessel van der Kolk's book *The Body Keeps the Score* explains it beautifully. When we're in survival mode, it's hard to think clearly and we see danger everywhere, putting us on high alert. The negative meanings we then create mean that, alongside this very stressful experience, we might blame ourselves or feel very angry at the world around us. This is hard enough to manage for anyone. What happens when there is also a brand new, very needy baby to deal with?

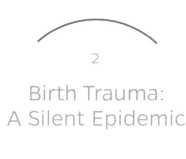

2

Birth Trauma:
A Silent Epidemic

Diagnosing birth trauma should be simple, shouldn't it? And, if someone has a difficult birth, then we should be offering them support in case they are traumatised, shouldn't we? But birth trauma is complex, and in many ways trauma after birth is very different from trauma after a different traumatic experience.

Imagine you and your partner had a serious road traffic accident, during which you had felt deeply concerned for your life. In the hospital, it is likely that people would ask you how you were feeling about the accident. They would check whether or not your partner was injured. Your GP might ask you if you had any symptoms of PTSD. Your friends and family members would be concerned, offering you practical support as well as emotional support.

Now imagine the same scenario, but this time you arrive at the hospital and everyone is concerned about your car. No one asks you how you're feeling, and your partner is ignored. And if you or your partner express any distress you are told 'But your car is OK! You should be so happy!' They're right, you do love your car. But then you have to get back in your car, and look at your car every day, and clean it, and people continually ask you about your car, and you put up photos of your car all over your home. And over time, you think, 'Well, I'm probably OK because I should be'. A year later, everyone comes together to celebrate your car accident and you just have to smile and try not to cry. And even though you can't face driving your car again, you just learn to take the bus.

Feeling traumatised after a birth is complicated because often you don't feel like you should be traumatised. You want to get on with the task of parenting your new baby, and put the birth behind you. You may feel traumatised by a birth which, on the surface, was fairly uncomplicated – so you don't feel justified in feeling the way you do. And no one else feels you should be traumatised either. Everyone else wants you to get on with the task of parenting too, and your own feelings quickly become secondary. Birth trauma is complicated because you have a new baby. That baby may remind you of the birth, complicating things further, but babies also have the habit of being enormously distracting. All of these things combine to create a recipe for avoidance. So that traumatic memory gets pushed aside, unless it is too difficult to ignore, or it is triggered in the form of a flashback or nightmare, or until you begin to plan a second pregnancy.

What is birth trauma?

There is, as yet, no formal definition for PTSD after birth, but there is growing recognition that people may feel traumatised by different aspects of pregnancy, birth and the postnatal period. Birth trauma is an incredibly new area of research – birth as a possible traumatic event was only recognised in research in the 2000s, and it wasn't until 2014 that birth was added to the list of traumatic events associated with the development of PTSD.

It's worth mentioning that most people are *not* traumatised after birth. Studies into PTSD after birth have suggested that it affects around 1 in 25 women, although many more may have some symptoms of trauma but not meet the full PTSD diagnostic criteria (15–45% of women rate some aspect of childbirth as traumatic, depending on the study you read). It is likely that the changes to the PTSD criteria in the DSM, with the removal of criterion A2 (as outlined in the previous chapter), may increase the rates of those diagnosed with PTSD after birth, as many may experience birth as 'a threat to the physical integrity of self or others' (criterion A1), but *not* respond to this with 'intense fear, helplessness, or horror' (criterion A2).

But half of women actually find birth an experience of growth (Ayers, 2017). The reason this is so relevant is because some of those women may have had a difficult experience of birth, yet come out of it feeling OK. So what is it that makes birth traumatic for some people and not for others?

What seems to be absolutely key to what makes one person's experience traumatic and another's positive, is the *subjective experience* of the birth. Cheryl Beck has talked about birth trauma as being 'in the eye of the beholder', and often being related to women feeling 'stripped of protective layers of caring': feeling uncared for at such a vulnerable time.

Why is birth trauma so hard to define?

As birth trauma is such a new area of study, many researchers and clinicians still find it difficult to define and thus discuss. You might have noticed this if you've attempted to speak to a friend, family member or healthcare professional who isn't understanding of birth trauma. Partly, this is because birth is usually not seen as a traumatic event, in the way that a road accident would be. People expect birth to be a powerful, positive experience. Or they acknowledge that it may be tough, but assume that you will feel amazing once you meet your baby. Or they think that it's just 'women's lot' – the God-given result of Eve's original sin – and therefore something we shouldn't complain about. It takes quite a mental shift to accept that some people find birth so traumatic that it can affect their mental health, their relationships and their view of the world. Unfortunately this situation creates a double whammy: you might be left feeling distressed, but unjustified in that distress, compounding it and adding shame into the mix.

Birth trauma is also complicated because it often exists alongside other mental health conditions such as postnatal depression (20–75% of people with PTSD after birth also have postnatal depression, depending on the study you read). Many of those who develop birth trauma and postnatal depression may also have experienced previous trauma (Sperlich, 2015) and have had symptoms of trauma already, which were not recognised. It is also hard to recognise what may be symptoms of trauma, and what might be part of a normal early parenting experience – for example, half of women who have *not* experienced traumatic births may have symptoms of hyperarousal; being very vigilant to the needs of your baby is also a healthy, helpful part of early bonding. So it can be very difficult for both you as a parent, and for a healthcare professional, to tease apart what is birth trauma, what is anxiety, what is postnatal depression and what is a normal part of adjusting to parenting.

It may also be that it was not the birth itself that was traumatic, but the events around the birth, such as your journey through pregnancy, the postnatal experience and feeding challenges. Birth trauma, then, comes to encompass many different things. Essentially, it relates to all psychological symptoms of trauma following birth and the circumstances around birth.

Do I have birth trauma?

Until very recently, the 'Impact of Events Scale' was most often used to diagnose PTSD after birth, but many of the questions on the scale are not appropriate to those who have given birth (for example, many parents experience sleep disturbance because they have a new baby who wakes a lot!). There are a couple of other measures which are used for birth trauma, but the newest measure (validated, appropriate to use with parents and created in line with the current DSM criteria) is the City Birth Trauma Scale (2018).

To be diagnosed with PTSD after birth, you would expect to have believed during your labour, birth or soon afterwards that either you or your baby were at serious risk of injury or death. You would then have at least one 're-experiencing' symptom, such as memories of the birth which feel outside of your control; at least one 'avoidance' symptom, such as trying to avoid thinking about the birth; at least two symptoms of negative thoughts or feelings, such as finding it hard to remember parts of the birth; and at least two symptoms of hyperarousal, such as feeling jumpy. You would expect to have had these symptoms for over one month, and for them to be affecting your daily life.

If you suspect that you do have some symptoms of trauma, please consider speaking to a healthcare or mental health professional who can help you access support.

Who gets birth trauma?

In the past 20 years, there has been a huge growth in research looking into birth trauma and who is most likely to feel traumatised by birth. Susan Ayers, a research psychologist who leads the Centre for Maternal and Child Health Research at City University, has been instrumental in adding to our understanding of the prevalence, causes and treatments of birth trauma. She has suggested a 'diathesis-stress model' of birth trauma, outlining the factors before pregnancy, during birth and in the postnatal period which can lead to PTSD and symptoms of trauma.

Before pregnancy

It doesn't take a psychologist to guess that having a history of abuse or trauma can make it more likely that you will find birth traumatic. Beck, Driscoll & Watson (2013) point out how re-traumatising birth can be for survivors of sexual abuse. Even the most common of interventions (such as internal examinations) can feel violating, and phrases such as 'just open your legs for me' can be triggering. The physical process of birth itself can also trigger traumatic memories, and if the body remains a source of shame then this can complicate both the pregnancy and the birth. It becomes more likely, then, that someone who has experienced sexual abuse prior to the birth may cope with this by dissociating, which itself makes post-traumatic stress symptoms more likely after the birth. Careful support and helping the woman or birthing person feel in control, prepared for the physical experience of birth and reassured throughout the antenatal and birth process can counter some of these difficulties.

A history of mental health problems, such as anxiety and depression, can also make birth more traumatic, as can a fear of birth, and 'poor coping strategies' (which are often linked to anxiety and depression too), such as avoidance. You can see how these might create a vicious cycle, where feeling anxious can increase your fear of birth, but using avoidance (e.g. not attending midwife appointments, or perhaps attending but not asking questions about the birth) can lead to feeling more out of control during the birth itself.

Having complications in pregnancy, or health problems (such as severe pre-eclampsia), can also increase the likelihood of finding birth traumatic. This may be due to the increased chance of needing intervention during birth, which (as outlined below) can lead to a traumatic experience.

There has been recognition that support in the antenatal period and during birth can counter some of these risks. It's also important to remember that having these experiences does not guarantee that your birth will be traumatic, and that, with support, birth can be a positive experience for you.

During birth

During birth, there are particular factors that can increase the chances that birth will be experienced as traumatic. These involve the birth itself, how you feel about it, and how you feel about the care you receive.

 Women who have birth complications and need intervention, or who have operative birth, are more likely to have symptoms of trauma afterwards. Some have suggested that an emergency C-section alone could be seen as a 'traumatic stressor', as this often includes an '*actual or threatened serious injury*' to the woman and/or the baby.

Feeling high levels of negative emotion has also been linked to symptoms of trauma after the birth; this may again be due to feeling out of control, frightened or helpless. Those who dissociate during birth (as with any other traumatic event) are also more likely to feel traumatised afterwards.

To me, the most crucial factor which can influence trauma during birth is the role of 'interpersonal factors' – how you relate to those around you. Research has shown time and time again that a low level of perceived support and feeling out of control are linked to PTSD. The way people are treated during birth is critical. Studies have suggested that a third of specifically distressing traumatic memories (known as 'hotspots' in CBT) are related to issues such as feeling abandoned, lacking in support or being ignored. If a professional is experienced as if they are a perpetrator then this is more likely to result in PTSD. You can also see how coercive language, such as 'You don't want to harm your baby, do you?' could in itself be seen as a traumatic stressor, leading to fear of injury to the baby.

A note on pain

It is a sad fact that women frequently have the experience of feeling that their pain – psychological or physical – is being downplayed or denied. This can affect how women feel during birth, how their pain is managed, and their recovery.

There is a growing body of research to suggest that women's experiences of pain are often taken less seriously than men's (although this is complicated depending on the gender of the assessor). The Birth Trauma Association has highlighted how this can impact on experiences of birth, with inadequate pain relief often cited as a factor leading to trauma in their BTA Charter. A recent US study also found that postnatal depression was more common in women who experienced greater levels of pain in the postnatal period – which indicates that women and birthing people may find that their physical symptoms are instead attributed to mental health difficulties.

Anya Hayes, pilates instructor and mothers' wellness expert, writes:

'I know that first time round I experienced a shocking amount of pain postnatally – which lasted for (I felt) a shocking amount of time (over a year) and wasn't taken seriously when I went to the GP several times to question whether my healing was normal – 'it's fine, it's all normal, you've had a baby, go away and stop being neurotic' (if not literally what was said, this was the take-home message).

I found out over a year later, during a birth debrief, that I had had an extra vertical incision made on my caesarean incision, in order to facilitate the speedy exit of my son in time to save his life. Therefore this 'extra' pain I was experiencing was entirely legitimate – and even knowing this rather than being fobbed off would have made a difference to my mental health and experience.

If you're being fobbed off when you're experiencing pain, that's going to take its toll on your mental health. This is a multi-layered issue of awareness and referral pathways and the general societal dismissal of women's issues. Postnatal health is a feminist issue. Even if that word turns you off, it IS. We need to learn to advocate for ourselves better, but it's distressing having to fight to be heard.'

Women often describe feeling that their concerns about their recovery are not taken seriously, leading to infection, or a need for intervention going unnoticed. Campaigns such as Pelvic Roar and the Pelvic Floor Patrol have highlighted how long women have been expected to accept pelvic floor dysfunction after birth.

Psychological pain is, of course, also denied. This was most recently demonstrated by stories in the media suggesting that women should not speak about their traumatic births, leading many to feel that their trauma was being silenced.

It may be that this is of particular note to women of black and ethnic minority backgrounds, with a number of studies suggesting a racial bias in assessments and treatment of pain.

After birth

Postnatally, other factors can lead to traumatic symptoms continuing. This might include additional stresses, unhelpful coping strategies (for example, dulling feelings by drinking alcohol) and poor support.

What can make trauma after birth so difficult to recover from, without specialist support, is continued 'triggers', such as birthdays, and the possibility of having another child (this latter point is discussed in Chapter 6). Beck (2006) has highlighted how difficult birthdays can be for those who have experienced birth trauma, both in the anxiety leading up to the birthday (the anniversary of the traumatic event), finding it hard to celebrate the day itself, and the fragility you might feel afterwards.

When your baby is ill

Sometimes the events surrounding your baby's birth can be what cause a traumatic response. Having a preterm baby has been strongly associated with developing PTSD. Although national guidance recommends all parents who have a child in a Neonatal Intensive Care Unit (NICU) should have access to psychological and social support, 30% of English neonatal units surveyed by the charity Bliss had no psychological support at all for parents. Bliss is campaigning for family-centred care in NICUs, as the frightening experience of giving birth to a baby who is unwell can also be compounded by the way that this is handled. Many talk about how their distress was exacerbated by being placed on a postnatal ward without their baby. Claud, one of the mums involved in the Make Birth Better campaign, describes her experience:

> *'I got to see him briefly before he was taken to NICU to be hooked up to antibiotics. My partner went with him of course and I was taken to a recovery ward. I felt fortunate but I did not feel like a mother.*

If I was a mother then where was my child?

If I was a mother then why couldn't I give my baby his first feed?

If I was a mother then why didn't my body work?

Morphine was doing its job and I should have welcomed its message to sleep. Instead, I was sat up in bed frantically trying to ensure I could produce milk and listening to the other new parents on the ward who had their children with them.

The importance of skin-to-skin is something that is hammered home at every antenatal class, alongside the bonding experience of the first feed. I didn't get to experience either of those things. My son was 50 metres down the corridor, alone, and this compounded my feeling of failure.'

The stress of looking after a baby in NICU can mean that it takes some months to recognise that you are struggling with symptoms of trauma. If this has been your experience, please do consider speaking to someone about it. Bliss offers a wide range of support for parents who have a baby who has been born prematurely or unwell.

When your baby dies

Following the death of a baby, it seems obvious that parents may suffer from a traumatic grief reaction, or from PTSD. It is perhaps surprising how little research there has been in this area, with some studies suggesting that making memories following the loss of a baby can reduce symptoms of trauma. This has been written into the NICE guidelines, which now recommend that parents whose baby is stillborn or dies soon after birth should be offered choices – such as seeing and holding the baby, seeing a photograph of the baby or creating mementos – alongside a trained facilitator. However, the charity SANDS (Stillbirth and Neonatal Death Society) has found that many Trusts do not have midwives trained in bereavement care, and less than half of Trusts and care boards have mandatory bereavement care training. This means that healthcare professionals may inadvertently respond to a bereavement in a way which could compound a traumatic response. Cheryl Titherly, of SANDS, says:

> 'The care bereaved parents receive following the death of their baby is crucial. Good care cannot remove parents' grief, but it can help them through this devastating time. There are many examples of excellent care across the country, however there are still very significant variations in the provision of bereavement care. SANDS is working to ensure that parents – whoever they are and whereever they are – can access the care they need when their baby dies.'

I spoke to fellow clinical psychologist Michelle Tolfrey, who experienced a stillbirth with her first daughter Orla and has spent the last three years raising awareness of the impact of baby loss. I asked her what can help parents after losing a baby:

> 'Losing a baby during pregnancy or after birth can be utterly devastating; your hopes and dreams shattered in one fell swoop. The feelings that arise are often confusing and overwhelming: sadness, anger, anxiety and jealousy can present with an intensity that you may never have experienced before. Things that never used to bother you can suddenly become terrifying and you may feel as though the person you thought you once were has gone forever. Grief following baby loss can be a lonely and isolating place. All of a sudden, there are babies and happy families everywhere you look, and the life that you were hoping for that has been cruelly ripped away seems to be taunting you.
>
> But you are not alone. What you are thinking is okay and normal and what you are feeling is important, and it matters. You might find solace in finding other people's stories

online: charity websites, blogs and social media are bursting with bereaved parents wanting to tell their story. Some may resonate, others less so, but that's okay – there is no right or wrong way to respond in the face of baby loss. Find platforms where you feel safe to connect with others, such as joining online forums and groups, following baby loss hashtags or attending local support groups. Find ways to talk about your baby and your experience to those you trust. Honour your baby in whichever way feels right for you: display photos and other keepsakes you may have, create a memory box, start a blog, fundraise, write their name, have a tattoo, find a special place that you can visit that brings you a feeling of connection with them – whatever feels comforting and comfortable for you.

Ensure that you focus on your own needs, both emotionally and physically. It is easy to forget that baby loss is a very physical experience and that your body needs time to recover too. Also remember that there is no set timeframe in grief and it can take a long time for the intense waves of sadness to lessen. Baby loss can change you considerably, in the same way that bringing a baby home can; however, you will find that aspects of the old you will start to return.

And finally, please don't try to survive this difficult time alone. Ask for help. Talk to your partner if you can. Take as much time as possible before returning to old activities, including work (although I appreciate that this has its own challenges). And please don't put pressure on yourself to feel or do anything – someone else's journey through loss is not yours, so try to respect what is arising within and for you.'

When you are from a minority group

While very little research has been done in this area, it makes sense that women and birthing people from minority communities may have a higher incidence of birth trauma. The National Maternity Survey (2010) found that women from Black and Minority Ethnic (BAME) communities, as well as those from poor backgrounds and women with physical and learning disabilities, were all less likely to feel that they had been treated with care and respect during their maternity journey, and were less likely to feel involved in their care decisions. Mothers from BAME and migrant communities both also reported poor communication and prejudiced staff attitudes. The impact of being from a black and minority ethnic community has been highlighted in the recent MMBRACE report, which found that black women are five times more likely and Asian women twice as likely to die compared to white women, and called for urgent research into the reasons for this.

Black women have themselves identified that their pain and concerns are often ignored – Candice Braithwaite, co-founder of Make Motherhood Diverse, said in a recent HuffPost article:

'I think we are long past putting this wholly deplorable outcome on pre-pregnancy health risks and social economic circumstances. It's time to say it like it is: this is happening due to racial bias. Since slavery the falsehood that black women can endure more pain than any other woman is a rhetoric which has been sold tirelessly'.

I asked Mars Lord, founder of Abuela Doulas (who runs a 'Reproductive Justice' retreat to highlight the need for equitable maternity services) how health services can redress this imbalance:

'With the release of the MMBRACE 2018 report it is clear that something needs to change. This changes when we all begin to clamour together, to raise our voices and raise

awareness. This is not about a blame game, but an honest opening of eyes to see where the shortcomings are. The holding up of a mirror and changing the view.'

When you are LGBTI+

It is telling that there is so little research into the experiences of gay people, same-sex couples and non-gender-conforming people and their involvement in maternity systems. However, the little research or discussion that there is in this area suggests that maternity systems tend to show a heteronormative bias, and that there is an increased chance of stigma throughout the pregnancy, birth and postnatal journey.

Dr Karen Gurney, clinical psychologist and psychosexologist, told me:

'The experience of having your identity, sexuality or family structure invalidated is not only homophobic, but can trigger memories of a whole lifetime of invalidation and invisibility for people who do not identify as heterosexual, at a time of (potential) trauma.

Trans and non-binary people experience transphobia in a range of settings, but possibly none more than maternity services. Experiences of being misgendered, treated like an 'interesting case' for students and trainees to learn from, the use of terminology around anatomy that triggers dysphoria or the use of inappropriate pronouns can all be experiences that trigger trans and non-binary peoples' already heightened minority stress.

The experience of not being respected by healthcare professionals at that moment would be difficult enough for most people, but it is important to remember that this experience, for LGBTQI+ people, is potentially connected to a lifelong experience of minority stress and so has particular resonance. We need to see systemic changes to the language we use when talking about birth parents and their partners (in training as well as on clinical forms, notes used and so on), and encourage people to think about the assumptions made about relationship set-ups. Prospective parents should be routinely asked which pronoun they prefer, and how they wish to be referred to. This applies to antenatal classes too, where small group work often separates by gender.'

When you have a disability

Much of the research into birth trauma and disabilities focuses on children left with long-term injury after birth. However, the literature on the treatment of women and birthing people with both physical and learning disabilities suggests that they will face increased difficulty during their maternity experience – which may increase the likelihood of a traumatic experience.

Erin E. Andrews, a US psychologist has written about her own experience as a congenital triple amputee. She says:

'I was less concerned about the effects of my disability, and more concerned about the attitudes of others toward my pregnancy. As a rehabilitation psychologist, I am well aware that women with disabilities face barriers to reproductive health and that social biases exist which portray women with disabilities as asexual, infertile, and incapable as mothers.'

She describes assumptions about pregnancies for disabled women as high risk, and highlights how physical changes during pregnancy can have an impact, depending on the type of disability. Research has shown that, while most women with physical disabilities report positive experience of maternity care, there is a need for improved communication and individualised care, and access can also be problematic.

In contrast, women with learning disabilities often report

difficulties throughout their maternity journey. Often faced with disapproval when they become pregnant, women with learning difficulties tend to find their maternity experience unsatisfactory, particularly around interpersonal experiences (Malouf et al., 2017).

Complex trauma

Women who face multiple disadvantages or complex social factors are often under-represented in national guidance, research and policy. Birth Companions, in joint research with the Revolving Doors Agency, defines women with multiple disadvantage as those experiencing factors such as: drug and alcohol misuse; are a recent migrant or have asylum-seeker status; are aged under 20; experience domestic violence; homelessness; current or historical trauma; mental health and personality disorders; no recourse to public funds; trafficked women; criminal justice involvement; financial needs; physical disability; current involvement with social services and a history of being looked after. The research suggests that those facing multiple disadvantage may find it harder to access services and that they, and their babies, have poorer outcomes as well as a 'deep mistrust' of services.

Trauma on to trauma

It is fair to say that trauma is not simple. For one person, trauma may have been caused by a difficult birth experience alone. For another, that birth experience may have compounded earlier traumas. For another, a straightforward birth experience may have become traumatising due to their postnatal experience. For yet another, the situation they are living in may be causing trauma too. Some people may have a severe traumatic reaction, which is not recognised by those around them. I spoke to Dr Rebecca Moore, my Make Birth Better co-founder and a perinatal psychiatrist who specialises in birth trauma. Becca often sees women and families who have suffered a severely traumatic response to their birth. She said:

'The impact of severe trauma is far too often missed, undetected or misdiagnosed. Women can end up suffering for years with distressing symptoms or clinical depression, anxiety or PTSD and there can be a lifelong impact on their sense of self, their relationship with partners and families and their ability to parent and connect with their babies or cope through subsequent pregnancies. Severe trauma needs to be assessed quickly and sensitively and rapid local free specialist treatment should be available to all for as long as they need it, as trauma takes time to heal and most generic services do not recognise or respond to this well enough at all.'

Writing this outline of all of the factors contributing to traumatic birth can make it sound a little like I'm putting together the ingredients of a recipe. But I really want to point out what these different factors *feel like* for the people experiencing them. For example, we know that it is more likely birth will feel traumatic if you have an experience of abuse in your past or present. But for some reason this isn't taken into account for *all* women or birthing people coming into contact with maternity services. Many researchers suggest that we should move towards trauma-informed maternity services, which are built on compassionate, consensual and respectful care. Considering the number of people who have experienced abuse – 1 in 5 people have a history of childhood maltreatment, 1 in 5 have been sexually assaulted as an adult and 1 in 5 have experienced severe physical violence in an intimate relationship (Seng, 2015) – it makes sense that we treat *all* those in maternity services as if they have had an experience of trauma at some time in their lives.

The role of healthcare professionals

Within all of these different factors contributing to trauma, the one thread that runs throughout is the importance of healthcare professionals. In antenatal care, labour and birth, and the postnatal period, having support can moderate all of these risk factors – essentially, having care and reassurance can prevent any of these leading to a traumatic reaction. However, in many cases staff not only do not prevent trauma from occurring, but may actually also be the cause of it. This may happen at an individual level, which is discussed throughout the rest of this book, but also at a service level.

Are services causing trauma?

There are many professionals working in maternity and birth who attribute a large part of the blame for physical and psychological birth trauma to the way in which birth has become increasingly intervention-focused in recent years. One recent study found that vaginal birth with no intervention within the NHS has dropped to 22% (RCM, 2016). Sheila Kitzinger, in her book *Birth Crisis*, describes the way in which the active management of labour, which began in the 1960s, meant that women began to lose control of their birth experience. Tina Cassidy, in *Birth: The surprising history of how we are born*, further outlines the history of birth and the ways in which medical interventions have often left women as passive recipients of care rather than active participants in their birth. The argument that this can cause iatrogenic harm (harm caused by medical intervention) is one which has been instrumental in changes to policy in recent years, with Trusts changing their policies on issues such as the timeline for cervical dilation, and reducing the pressure to labour to a particular deadline. In the UK, both the National Institute for Health and Care Excellence (NICE, 2014) and Better Births

(2016) have highlighted the need for compassionate, person-centred care, which enhances both the woman's control and her subjective experience. There has also been international recognition, in documents such as the World Health Organization's 2018 recommendations on 'Intrapartum Care for a positive childbirth experience', that birth and care around birth should be woman-centred, stating:

> 'There has been a substantial increase over the last two decades in the application of a range of labour practices to initiate, accelerate, terminate, regulate or monitor the physiological process of labour, with the aim of improving outcomes for women and babies. This increasing medicalisation of childbirth processes tends to undermine the woman's own capability to give birth and negatively impacts her childbirth experience.'

Both the Maternity Transformation Programme and the WHO report outline similar recommendations, such as respectful care, continuity of carer and fully informed consent.

However, despite these policy statements, there has been an *increase* in intervention. Inductions are on the rise, from 20.3 to 29.3% in the last 10 years, which has been attributed to an increase in obesity, an increase in average maternal age and a drive to reduce the risk of stillbirth. Clearly reducing the stillbirth rates in the UK, among the highest in high-income countries, is crucial – but the experience of the woman must also be taken into account if such an increase in intervention is not also going to lead to an increase in birth trauma. It seems that there may be a vicious cycle being created, with increased intervention leading to increased birth trauma, which raises fear of childbirth, leading to an even greater risk of intervention and birth trauma.

Often it seems that, although evidence and policy point towards person-centred models of care, the realities of maternity services can prevent this. This has been exemplified recently by the contrast between a recent Cochrane review, which found that perineal massage and warm compresses could reduce third- and fourth-degree tears, and the Royal College of Obstetricians and Gynaecologists' Obstetric Anal Sphincter Injury care bundle, which did not include these methods due to a lack of standardisation and differences between teams. Instead, the more invasive 'Finnish grip' was recommended. It is telling that there is little data on women's views on these different interventions.

One thing that is clear about birth is that there is a huge difference in opinion about the best way to 'manage' it. You only need to spend a minute on Twitter to see how passionately these things are argued. But actually, when the woman or birthing partner and their family is placed firmly at the centre of the planning process, it doesn't really matter how others think birth should be managed. All that matters is what that family think, and how this is achieved in collaboration with the professionals around them.

Birth and the 'bad mother'

Before I finish this chapter, I would like to talk about how powerful stories of birth and motherhood can be, and the ways in which this can exacerbate a traumatic birth.

There is a narrative around birth, of the 'perfect birth', which is viewed almost as a marker of success. I've heard referrals to a 'gold standard' of birth – which is usually a natural, home water birth. Of course there are other idealised narratives too – that of the mother who will find breastfeeding easy, or the mother who fits into her size 10 jeans a fortnight after birth, or the mother who manages to keep her relationship exciting. These stories create an impossible standard, meaning that anything less than this can feel like a huge failure. Added to this is an idea that we must not speak about our fears or anxieties about birth. That we must only think positively, and this will mean our birth is positive. This results in feelings of shame if birth has not gone well. Perhaps it was because we were too anxious and stopped the natural birth process? We blame ourselves, or sometimes we blame the 'natural childbirth movement', rather than the many complex factors which we now know can cause birth to be difficult.

The distance between the realities of motherhood and these ideals has been talked about in depth in feminist analyses of birth and motherhood. Paula Nicolson, in her book *Postnatal Depression*, describes the difference between the myth of motherhood – that mothers are powerful and that motherhood is a natural, easy endeavour – and women's everyday experiences, in which they may feel invisible, exhausted and stressed. This, to me, is very relevant to the narratives we have around birth too. As Nicolson writes '*This means that the accompanying stresses of motherhood [and, I would add, birth] may be experienced by women as their own inadequacies*'. Women not only feel disappointed about their birth, but also that they should not be distressed, that they 'should' be coping and conforming to these ideals.

The resulting shame in having an imperfect birth, and thus becoming an imperfect mother, can hugely compound the experience of trauma. It feels as though your birth was your personal failure, and your continued distress means that you are continuing to 'fail'. This makes it very hard to admit to how difficult you might be finding things, so the trauma is left unresolved.

The general literature about trauma has highlighted how much shame can add to the distress caused by trauma. If you suffer from PTSD or symptoms of trauma, self-critical and self-attacking thoughts can actually feel like a current threat, exacerbating the symptoms. This seems to be particularly pertinent when you have experienced traumatic birth, when you may have not only self-critical thoughts, but also hear actual criticism from those around you, who minimise your distress. Conversely, if you are able to speak to yourself in warm and kind ways, you are more resilient to stressful and traumatic situations. Compassion-focused therapies can help to target such self-critical and shaming thoughts and ideas. You will find more information on therapies and recovery techniques in Chapter 5, but I wanted to share one exercise here which can help to develop self-warmth and soothing, called 'The Perfect Nurturer' (Lee, 2015).

The Perfect Nurturer

Imagine someone – or something – that would act as your perfect nurturer. They would care completely about your welfare, would be completely committed to help you and to take joy in your wellbeing, can endure your distress completely and are totally warm and accepting of you. They are infinitely wise, and strong. You might think of a person, a character from a book or film, or it might be someone imaginary. It might even be something more fluid, like an angel, a spirit or mythical figure.

Take some time to get your perfect nurturer firmly fixed in your mind. What do they look like? What does their voice sound like? Do they have a smell you can associate with them? Really try and get them fixed in your mind.

When you are thinking self-critical or shaming thoughts you can call on your perfect nurturer. Ask yourself what they might say if they heard you speaking to yourself in this way. What might they do to help you? How would they respond? In a difficult memory such as your birth, how would they protect you and reassure you?

In this way, you can practice knowing what it feels like to develop a kind and warm internal voice.

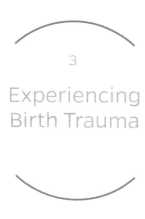

3

Experiencing
Birth Trauma

Slowly, slowly there is increasing recognition that birth trauma happens, and that it affects women and their families in complex ways. This recognition has come about partly due to the work of researchers and clinicians, who have highlighted the existence of PTSD and the experience of traumatic symptoms after birth. But mainly awareness has grown through the brave and tireless work of parents who have been through traumatic births themselves.

Hearing the voices of women and their partners not only enables professionals to learn from their experience to inform their own practice, but also helps those who have been through traumatic birth feel less alone. You might feel ashamed following a traumatic birth experience, and somehow to blame. Hearing the voices of others who have been through similar experiences shows us all that these experiences are *not* normal, *not* acceptable and *not* our fault.

During Birth Trauma Awareness week 2017, I invited women to send me their birth stories. I received 75 and analysed these (using a grounded theory methodology) to pull out the key themes. This chapter will describe these themes in brief, fitting them in with wider research. You can read more about the findings of the campaign and the sub-themes at www.makebirthbetter.org, where you will also find a lot of information about birth trauma and UK services.

The findings of the campaign reflected other research into women's experience of traumatic birth. There is now a growing body of qualitative research outlining the key themes emerging for women after a traumatic birth. In 2010, Elmir and colleagues summarised qualitative research into birth trauma and identified six major themes, which closely link to the themes identified here:

- Feeling invisible and out of control
- To be treated humanely
- Feeling trapped
- The reoccurring nightmare of my childbirth experience
- A rollercoaster of emotions
- Disrupted relationships
- A strength of purpose: a way to succeed as a mother

Theme 1: A Force Bigger than Me – the physical process of birth

'The strength of being a woman is truly awesome.' L.P.

When birth was positive for women (often this was second time around), many of the stories described how surprising the physical process of birth was. For those women who experienced positive births, this left them feeling awed by how their bodies worked. Such experiences enabled women to not only feel positive about their birth, but also well prepared for the challenges of early parenthood. This reflects research into

The Power I Felt

A FORCE BIGGER
THAN ME

You're Being Violated

All I cared about was the
safety of the baby (fear)

The Physical Impact

The Care Never Comes

They're Overstretched

HEROES AND
VILLAINS

I will never forget

He was literally my hero

Out of my mind

DELIVERY INTO
PARENTHOOD

Something truly terrible

I had no idea

I HAD
NO IDEA

Stop making a fuss

Missing out on baby

Tainted pregnancies

Impact on partner

What pregnant women
need to know

MAKE BIRTH
BETTER

What professionals
need to know

The secret shame

Nowhere to turn

Talking really does help

What providers
need to know

What we all
need to know

Themes and sub-themes of the Make Birth Better campaign

parenting self-efficacy, which suggests that a positive birth experience closely correlates with parenting confidence and competence (Bryanton et al., 2008).

In contrast, the women who described feeling shocked were left feeling uncertain and shaken about their capacity to cope. For a number of the women in the campaign, this was due to physical or medical complications that sometimes led to long-lasting injury. For some, this included fear that they were close to death during their labour.

'The consultant looked like something out of a horror film – neck to foot plastered in blood – which didn't phase me at the time because I was convinced I was going to die and, sadly, I actually wanted to.' J.B

For a proportion of women, this extended to pain caused by the actions of healthcare professionals. There were a number of descriptions of both coercive language and actual physical violation.

'If I was an alcoholic, soldier, an anorexic, there would be a dedicated team who could help me, but the truth is that there is nowhere to turn for birth trauma. If I'd been raped, I'd be referred to a specialist, but in my eyes, it's comparable to a rape – you're being violated, down in that area, and that is never going to be the same again.' J.P.

Understandably, when feeling so out of control and disempowered, women also described not knowing whether their babies would come out of the experience harmed. Often, women were afraid for the baby's life. There were babies who were born unwell and taken to NICU, and women described not knowing – sometimes for prolonged periods of time – whether or not their babies were alive. Out of the 75 stories I received, one mother had experienced a late-term loss. This was, in fact, not a traumatic experience for her due to the incredible support she received at the time. However, the fear of loss was present in many of the stories.

'It all feels a little hazy now but I remember how devastated and helpless I felt, I was convinced at this point that I'd lost my baby.' S.S.

'I came round an hour after he was born, to be told I'd been "asleep". At that point I had no idea whether he had been born, whether he was alive.' F.C.

A word on obstetric violence

As of writing, there was no agreed-upon global definition of obstetric violence – a controversial term which I've seen frequently cause 'heated debate' in discussions about birth. Definitions encompass clear violations such as assault, intervention without consent and coercion. Some have also argued that the way that services are structured, with 'factory line conditions' (Lokugamage & Pathberiya, 2017), which follow protocol over a clear evidence base and individualised care, is also a form of obstetric violence. In this sense, others have suggested that we should move away from only examining individual experiences, and look more fully at the structural dimensions of obstetric violence – the social and cultural factors which maintain it – in order to more fully address it (Pickles, 2017).

Bohren and colleagues (2015) conducted a review of research into obstetric violence, and propose a typology for services to use as a definition. They suggest obstetric violence includes the following domains:

- physical abuse (for example, slapping or pinching during delivery);
- sexual abuse;
- verbal abuse such as harsh or rude language;
- stigma and discrimination based on age, ethnicity, socioeconomic status, or medical conditions;
- failure to meet professional standards of care (for example, neglect during delivery);
- poor rapport between women and providers, including ineffective communication;
- lack of supportive care, and loss of autonomy;
- health system conditions and constraints such as the lack of the resources needed to provide women with privacy.

Using this typology, each of the difficult birth stories I read during the campaign meets at least one of these criteria.

Whether or not it is labelled 'obstetric violence', it is clear that the actions of healthcare providers can be instrumental in causing or preventing birth trauma. Reed et al. (2017), in a worldwide survey, found that 66.7% of women saw healthcare providers' actions as instrumental to their birth trauma. Examples included ignoring mothers' knowledge of their own bodies and needs, coercion ('the dead baby card') and overt violation including examples of women being held down for interventions they did not consent to.

Theme 2: Heroes and Villains

The second theme focused on the vital influence of others, and was incredibly polarised. Healthcare professionals were seen as either neglectful and/or abusive, or as saviours. Perhaps this is inevitable given the huge amount of research that has highlighted the role of healthcare professionals, particularly midwives, in defining a person's maternity experience. A number of studies have demonstrated that quality in the relationship between a mother and her midwife can promote a positive birth experience (Dahlberg & Aune, 2013), even down to the way language is used (Mobbs et al., 2018).

Where staff were helpful and supportive, they were referred to as 'superheroes', having the potential to turn a difficult experience into a manageable one. Feeling safe and being treated with kindness seemed to be especially important here, with staff being praised for these qualities.

'I was well supported and encouraged to allow things to unfold at their own pace. I felt held and safe and had a peaceful birth with an incredibly swift recovery' S.W.

When staff were not caring, or were coercive, pressuring, rude or aggressive, this was clearly frightening. What was apparent from the stories was that staff inattention (frequently caused by understaffing, which women were aware of and tried to be forgiving about) felt deeply abandoning. When we think of pregnancy and birth as being a time when women often feel very vulnerable, it is understandable that feeling contained and cared for becomes essential.

Considering the current shortage in maternity units of both midwives and doctors, as recognised by the Royal College of Midwives and the Royal College of Obstetricians and Gynaecologists, this is in danger of becoming a pipe dream rather than the baseline it should be. The role of healthcare professionals in influencing a woman's feelings about her birth cannot be overstated; one recent research study suggested that two-thirds of women attributed the cause of their birth trauma to the actions of healthcare professionals (Reed et al., 2017).

'I am extremely thankful for the NHS, and painfully aware of the struggles the staff face, however, it was my aftercare where things really went wrong. I was unwell following my C-section, I was given high doses of painkillers, iron tablets and pretty much ignored. I didn't bond with [my baby], I was exhausted (as all new mothers are), I was distant, and if I'm honest, most of it is a blur.... All I remember is how frightened and alone I felt, I felt as though I was detached from my body, but still feeling the pain, I felt so weak and lifeless, and no one listened.' L.B.

I had expected upon reading the stories that partners too would be hailed as heroes, alongside staff. While this was certainly the case, more often they seemed helpless, ignored and left suffering with their own trauma, as discussed more fully in Chapter 3.

'My partner said afterwards it was one of the worst things he has ever seen in this life.... It only takes one smell, a noise and I am instantly transported back, it also had an impact on my partner. When discussing future children, it was always brought up – what if it happens again? We had to come to accept that the birth of my son was one of the worst times of my life.' V.C.

Theme 3: Delivery into Parenthood

This theme described the wide-ranging ways in which birth had an impact on women, both in their own psychological symptoms, and the impact on the baby and their partner.

Some of the women writing had received diagnoses of PTSD, but most had not. They described a range of symptoms, many fitting with traumatic stress such as flashbacks, nightmares and hypervigilance. This sometimes extended to others around them, such as worry about their baby's health. Some women also described low mood and suicidal thoughts. These were described not as a sudden onset, but as a slow realisation that something quite fundamental had changed for them. This could be a sense of failure or feeling deeply damaged, a feeling that remained with women for months and years after the birth.

This is not uncommon with symptoms of trauma, which can develop months after the event. One study (Garthus-Niegel et al., 2015) explored PTSD symptoms after birth in women two years postnatally and found a proportion of women who had new PTSD symptoms that had not been present at 8 weeks post-partum. This is significant as, of course, at this time women often aren't regularly seeing healthcare professionals they can discuss these symptoms with.

'I think women need time. After my first birth, whilst it was traumatic at the time being stitched, it was such a relief to have a baby after my awful pregnancy and then they are so all consuming, it wasn't until about six months later that I realised I wasn't actually happy…. I think a lot of birth trauma, difficulties… probably go unreported for this reason'. A.C.

Symptoms were often associated with feelings of guilt and inadequacy, linked both to the birth itself and missing out on the experience of early motherhood they had expected. Many women described feeling cheated out of the 'crucial first moments' due to either their own physical state, or because their babies had been taken to NICU.

'They put him next to my head after what felt like forever. I thought "I don't know you. You're not what I expected". Then I threw up. The birth really was ok, as these things go, but that reaction felt so horribly far from what I "should" have felt. That blissful first eye contact. I was sure I'd missed this essential chance to bond.' V.N.

It is almost inevitable that this creates a rupture in the early mother–baby relationship. Many mothers – not just those who have experienced a traumatic birth – describe feeling disappointed that they didn't feel besotted with their newborn. This is a myth that remains very powerful. Yet we have known since 1962 that the majority of mothers do not feel that rush of love upon first seeing their children. In fact, in that 1962 study by Newton and Newton, only about a quarter did, with over 10% feeling 'indifferent' or 'disgusted'… and it will come as no surprise that those with positive feelings after birth reported a better relationship and better care during birth than those with more rejecting feelings.

Where the traumatic experience can cause difficulties in that early relationship, though, is through the feeling of detachment many women experience. This can be seen as a symptom of the trauma – either through disassociation, where you might feel distant from the world or even from your own body, or through avoidance. When the baby represents a reminder of the trauma you have been through, it makes sense that you might feel detached from him or her. Of course, the guilt that this then creates in women who are already feeling ashamed after their birth experience can cause huge distress and make it even less likely they will seek support.

'I struggled to bond with my baby, I couldn't breastfeed him, I felt like someone had given me somebody else's three-month-old giant baby, I was underweight, anaemic and probably a bit traumatised but for whatever reason, I smiled to everyone and anyone, acted like I was just happy that I got to go home with my baby and didn't blink an eyelid at the lack of support I felt after getting home. … I am surrounded by people who constantly talk like they have accomplished more because they gave birth naturally and breastfed and I'm ashamed to say it does make me feel like less of a mother or less of a woman.' S.H.

As mentioned, the impact on partners was often in leaving them feeling vicariously traumatised. However, there was also the added impact of changes to the couple relationship. For some couples, the experience also created a barrier between them with both parties shell-shocked and unable to process it together. When dealing with the stresses of a new baby, which place enormous stress on any couple's relationship, processing a traumatic birth adds a layer of complexity and distress. This has an impact on a couple's feelings about subsequent pregnancies. For some, going through pregnancy and birth again feels impossible, a theme which has been repeated in previous research (e.g. Iles and Pote, 2015), which has also found that women may have fewer children after a difficult birth, and wait for longer before becoming pregnant again (Gottvall and Waldenstrom, 2002). For those who did go on to have second children, the level of support received after a traumatic first birth actually meant that many second births felt like healing experiences. Again, this is reflected in previous research (Beck and Watson, 2010), which showed that 75% of women found their second birth an improvement. Where this does not happen, however, it can feel like a double failure and worsen symptoms of trauma. Those women who do go on to have subsequent births may also make decisions related to their traumatic experience, such as choosing a home birth or freebirth over a hospital birth (Reed at al., 2017). This is discussed in more detail in Chapter 6.

Theme 4: I Had No Idea

Women spoke about a pressure to 'cope' and a lack of awareness of how birth could impact upon them, from antenatal education through to the postnatal period. This was both in a lack of open and honest information given prior to birth, and messages after birth that their feelings were not acceptable.

Antenatal education is a tricky dilemma, and educators need to find a balance between providing information and not raising anxiety. Many women feel that, in fact, they only hear negative birth stories (one of the key reasons why the Positive Birth Movement was created by Milli Hill six years ago). This, however, does not seem to be reflected in antenatal education nor in wider stories about birth, leaving women feeling ill-informed about how birth could be.

'I was riled by the misconception and false representation of birth (severe sleep deprivation, pain and post-birth hormones didn't help). If we believe Hollywood and Hollyoaks *then we rush to hospital when our waters break and give birth shortly afterwards. Obviously this is not a depiction of reality, but it feeds into expectations. For many people expectations of birth are vastly different to the reality they experience. It's not just TV that contributes to these expectations, often as a society we do not talk about when things go wrong or when birth is traumatic. Maybe we are scared of making other people anxious? Whatever the reason, as a result people often feel unable to speak about their difficult birth experiences or seek help when needed.'* E.M.

At Make Birth Better, we often hear from women who feel that their antenatal education was not adequate, while simultaneously hearing about Trusts in which antenatal education has been cut or is being provided at a cost. It is remarkable how many women feel set up to fail. This may, of course, not only reflect antenatal education and wider social messages, but also the inability of services to provide the care necessary for a positive birth experience. Clients I have met throughout my career – both in therapy and in groups – often remark on how lost they feel in early pregnancy. All the onus is on us to find out about birth and educate ourselves but, as the old adage goes, 'you don't know what you don't know'. In the absence of a trusted person to guide us through, women are often left feeling that they are completely unprepared for birth.

'So the drip, I had the pethidine injection to start with, I knew nothing about this, pain relief wasn't discussed in my appointments, I wasn't told to "inform myself" of my options either. Not that it would have helped anyway, how do you look for something when you don't know what you're looking for?'
A.B.

This continues during birth itself, if staff do not inform women and their partners about what is happening and why. Many women also described feeling particularly shocked at what happened after birth. This might have been as simple as partners being told to go home, when mothers were still reeling from their experience. Or, for some, the experience of NICU or further physical complications for themselves.

'However, the birth being frightening is minor in my head compared to how I was spoken to and treated on the postnatal ward. I named and shamed during my complaint to the hospital and I was assured the midwives in question were going to be dealt with. The one incident that really gets to me is one day I laid on my bed sobbing. I'd closed my curtain so as not to draw attention. A midwife came in and told me to open my curtain and asked what I was "making a fuss" about. I told her my baby was in intensive care (heartbreaking when everyone else on the ward had their baby by their bed) and I was just feeling a bit sad today. Plus I'd been living in a hospital bay for four weeks at this point and was just feeling claustrophobic and like I was going out of my mind. Instead of being kind or sympathetic, she told me to "pull myself together", yanked my curtain across and left me to it. In that moment, I felt like the *most scared, pathetic person in the world and can definitely say it triggered, maybe not postnatal depression as such, but very serious "baby blues".* Z.D.

Running beneath these experiences was the common thread of being dissuaded, implicitly or explicitly, from talking about how difficult the birth and aftermath had been. Women often then blamed themselves for feeling this way – coming to the conclusion that there was something wrong with them, rather than being angry at those around them. This led to their feelings being buried even deeper. Partly this can be viewed as another symptom of traumatic stress – avoiding reminders and feelings associated with the birth. Focusing on looking after the newborn allowed women to do this. But expectations of how things should be after birth also exacerbated these feelings – women spoke of feeling ashamed at how different their experience was to their ideas of early motherhood:

'It needs to be talked about. Too many mums feel like failures before they even start and too many mums slip into PND by not being open about how they feel. There is a stigma around how we should be feeling and how amazing, magical and beautiful the whole experience is supposed to be... even the slightest deviation from that and we clam up, not wanting to be judged or criticised, we just say "it's fine" and struggle on.' A.W.

Implicit in many of the stories was women's fear of how they would be judged if they spoke about their feelings. This brings me back to the concern many mums have of frightening other women who have not yet had their babies, but again demonstrates just how strong that cultural message is that birth – and motherhood – should be enjoyable, and when it is not that represents a failure of the woman rather than the systems and culture around her.

The stigma associated with this pervades so much of perinatal mental health work. A number of studies (e.g. Button et al., 2017; NCT 'Hidden Half' campaign) have shown that less than half of women struggling with their mental health during pregnancy or after birth will seek help (and even then, many women who are brave enough to speak to someone about their experience won't access the support they need). This was reflected in the stories – women described a cycle in which they were worried about seeking help, their treatment at the hands of NHS staff made them even more reluctant to seek help, and when they did try to seek help it was not forthcoming.

'Nobody ever offered to talk to me about it. About how they started administering the anaesthetic and barking at me to lie down before my husband in another room had his scrubs on. How they didn't pass on the message about how nervous I was and would like to be talked through the procedure and have the radio on, that I even had a playlist on an Ipod. How nobody spoke to me throughout or explained what was going on, but how the surgeon bollocked his team for letting the placenta fall on the floor ("somebody clear this bloody mess up") or bringing the wrong size dressing. How nobody comforted me when I started to shake and haemorrhage and vomit while I was being stitched up. How nobody bothered to tell me if the baby was healthy and didn't even show me his face for a good five minutes after he was born. How they let me fall asleep on the first night with a half-dressed baby on the bed between my legs because I was so weak I couldn't get him back into the crib and nobody came when I rang the buzzer. How they left me naked, unwashed and covered in day-old blood by an open door for the Bounty woman to wander in uninvited and dozens of passing visitors to see me at my most vulnerable. There it is again: "At least you have a healthy child".

You're encouraged to believe that as long as you have a healthy baby that nothing else matters. Of course, that's what matters most to me. And he is healthy and he is happy and he's loved and he's everything I could ever hope for. But there's absolutely no reason why that should be at the expense of my wellbeing.' B.

A word on stigma

Despite all the awareness-raising campaigns, social media hashtags and improved access to psychological therapies that have occurred in recent years, there remains enormous stigma for people in being open about their mental health problems.

Perhaps this is particularly profound in perinatal mental health, when parents are up against the contrast between their expectations and reality (which in itself increases feelings of guilt and shame). Parenting also invites such judgement from others, that many parents are deeply afraid that if they are open about their experience their children will be removed from them. One study found that 80% of women surveyed would find it difficult to disclose their mental health difficulties to a healthcare provider due to worries about stigma (Moore et al., 2017).

This isn't helped by the current culture of both the NHS and Child Services, where staff are working under such pressure that families are often not given the time and reflection that they deserve. There is such an enormous funding gap in Children's Services at present that many families (perhaps wisely) avoid seeking support knowing that help may not be available.

Alongside stigma, there does remain a lack of understanding about perinatal mental health. Many women report being misdiagnosed with postnatal depression after a traumatic birth, and men are often not screened for perinatal mental health problems.

One of the benefits of social media has been the increased discussion of mental health online. Such discussions can not only reduce stigma, but also challenge some of the assumptions we make about mental health – such as the idea that you can't have a mental health problem and be a good mother (Moore et al., 2016).

Sometimes such discussions – either online or with a friend or family member – can provide a stepping stone to seeking the help you need, and the confidence to try again if you don't get a good response the first time. If you are thinking about seeking support, do consider asking others about their experience in the Birth Trauma Association peer support group, or take a look at the map on the Make Birth Better website, which shows different services around the UK. You could also ask a question on our social media, and take a look at *How to Heal a Bad Birth*.

When women did manage to speak to a professional about their experiences, this was portrayed as very positive. Some women had birth debrief or Birth Reflections sessions with their local Trust, others spoke to peers or birth professionals, and some had psychological therapy or a combination of many different approaches. What seemed to be key was the feeling of being really heard, which both validated the severity of their experience and shifted that pervasive feeling of self-blame. There were women who felt, however, that no service had really been able to provide the support they needed. It is perhaps of note that many of the women with positive experiences of therapy had chosen to pay for private help to ensure they got the support they wanted – not an option which is possible for many.

'There is an upside (apart from my son obviously). It led me to becoming a doula. I hoped I could support women at this life-changing time so they could have a better experience than me, so they could feel empowered into motherhood. This helped me to go on my own long and explorative journey where I got to debrief my first birth with many different amazing women and I also got to see it in different ways from different perspectives. Even now writing this I feel more removed from it than I ever have. Time really is a great healer, if you seek help.

Before my second pregnancy, I needed help. I knew I couldn't experience that level of anxiety again. I went to the GP, explained I didn't want drugs and luckily, without question, he referred me for some CBT sessions. In just four magical sessions, my symptoms came way down and I got signed off. Two weeks later I found out I was pregnant.

I took everything I learned from my first birth into my second. I read, I reflected, I attended births as a doula, I hired a doula and I realised IT WAS ALL MY CHOICE. EVERYTHING. I also realised my feelings, my instinct, should not be underestimated. I WAS EMPOWERED.

I put the work in. I went there. To those difficult hard to reach places of vulnerability, shame, guilt, anger, sadness, grief and I processed and unpicked them, let them be and then did my best to let them go. It wasn't easy but it was very necessary to move on and into my next birth.' Jenna

Theme 5: Make Birth Better

During the campaign, women and birth professionals were asked to include their thoughts on what would 'make birth better' in their stories. I divided these into messages applicable throughout the maternity journey: for pregnant women and their partners, maternity professionals and wider society. These reflected many of the themes already described, the need for pregnant women to be better informed about all of the different possible outcomes in birth, to be granted as much support and reassurance as possible during birth, and to seek help after a difficult birth if necessary.

This extended to very clear suggestions for birth professionals too, again prior to, during and after birth. These centred around encouraging women to be informed of different possible outcomes and aspects of birth, but also underlined the need for women to feel respected during birth. Women spoke frequently about simply needing more time. As I will discuss more fully in Chapter 7, this is something that not only needs to be heard by healthcare professionals, but healthcare providers and commissioners. As well as by all of us. Being prepared to give women time to explore their hopes and fears for birth, to support maternity professionals to do this, and to be open to discussing birth stories without offering platitudes would in itself go a long way to improving women's experiences of birth.

> 'What would make birth better? Time. Everything felt so rushed. I saw seven different midwives and it took hours to get pain relief. I think if midwives have the time to support, listen and care for a woman in labour whether she is 1cm dilated or 10.
>
> But yes... just more time would have been wonderful. After the birth too. You need someone to sit, listen and talk you through. Maybe offer a hand squeeze and a cuppa too. I had that time but eight months after birth with a wonderful midwife from the supervisors of midwives who talked me through my hospital notes and gave me a copy. She spent three hours at my house and was amazing! The nightmares stopped after that.' L.

If you've had the experience of being left to cope alone with the aftermath of a difficult birth, you may also have felt the impact of this on your partner and the rest of your family.

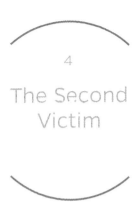

4

The Second Victim

A traumatic birth creates a ripple effect which impacts upon everyone in your circle – from your partner, to the medical professionals involved in the birth, your baby and the other people around you.

The concept of the 'second victim' was coined by Albert Wu (2000) in describing the impact of medical error on the doctor as well as the patient. Birth is one of the unique circumstances in which many people might be involved (you, your baby and your partner, as well as any medical professionals), so there are many 'second victims'. While they might not have been through the physical experience of a difficult birth, they are often left with symptoms of trauma and a double bind in which they feel discouraged from talking about their experiences.

I also wonder if, as a society, we are traumatised by birth. We see birth 'horror stories' in the news, unrealistic images of birth in film and TV, even the sharing of dramatic and shocking birth stories that we hear while sitting on our mothers' laps – all of these things have created an idea that birth is, at best, something to endure and, at worst, something we may not survive.

Trauma in partners

As the research on birth trauma is still a relatively new field, research about partners is clearly limited. Generally, it has focused on male partners, and numbers have been small. But some key themes have emerged that paint a picture of partners as being pushed aside during birth, ignored after birth and encouraged to diminish their feelings throughout.

Why have we ignored partners?

It's a relatively recent phenomenon that partners are invited into the birth room with us at all, with some hospitals keeping them on the other side of the doors until the 1980s. Even 40 years later, the presence of male partners is still debated. The well-known obstetrician Michel Odent has described the ways in which men can actually hinder birth, suggesting that women are best supported in a quiet, women-only environment with only a midwife present. It's also difficult to include partners in discussions about birth – even when they are invited to antenatal appointments, it's often difficult for both partners to take time off work or away from other children.

> *'When we spoke about it afterwards I didn't realise how much that had affected him! He said he felt useless in that moment to see them wheel me away and hear me screaming and there was nothing he could do, so he just started to get my belongings together from in the labour room until he was sent for, he thought that was going to be last time he saw us. Even though he arrived ok into the world that whole experience has been tainted for us both.'* A.W.

For some couples, pregnancy can be the first time in a relationship that gender roles suddenly become relevant and, while women are invited into an exclusive 'mum squad' in antenatal classes and courses, there is often not the equivalent support for their partners. For same-sex parents and parents who do not conform to traditional gender norms, there is even less available and they have the added burden of stigma to contend with.

Postnatal mental health problems in partners have only been acknowledged in the last 20 years or so (and even then often in inverted commas). Historically, mental health problems during pregnancy and postnatally have been seen as a medical condition, caused by neurochemical imbalances brought on by the physical changes of pregnancy and parenthood. So until very recently it was not thought possible that you could be affected if you hadn't been through the physical changes of pregnancy and birth. Now there is increasing awareness that perinatal mental health can be affected by a number of holistic factors, including physical changes, but also including social, cultural and personal circumstances. It has become clear that both parents can be affected.

On the few occasions that perinatal mental health in fathers has been researched, there's a chance that problems may have been missed. Many postnatal measures have not been validated for use with men, and a study in 2000 found that men require a lower cut-off when screening for postnatal depression (they need a score of 5/6 to be diagnosed with postnatal depression or anxiety, while in mothers this would be 7/8) (Matthey et al., 2000).

Further, problems in dads have often been linked either to postnatal depression in their partner, or to how it affects men's ability to 'provide support for their wives' (Areias et al., 1996). This implies that the man's role in birth and childrearing is to cope and to provide for their partners, rather than feel any impact themselves. You can see why men might be reluctant to talk about their own difficulties.

> '*I knew in my heart I wasn't bonding with M… I felt so torn between him and my wife's health and needs. I felt like I was searching all the time for how to prioritise when the reality was I didn't need to. I finally crashed one evening when chatting to my wife on the sofa and it became very apparent that I needed to seek some help. I had done what sadly many men do in situations like this. I was being tough and strong for my family and "not wanting to seem weak"'.* P.W.

How are partners affected?
Despite the continued debate about whether partners should even be present at birth, the vast majority of partners are keen to be in the birthing room and mothers and birthing people also feel that this is a crucial element of their own feeling of wellbeing. For many of us, the thought of *not* having our partner there at the baby's arrival (when usually they were there at its creation!) seems unthinkable.

However, even in a straightforward birth, partners can be stunned by the physical process we go through. Mark Harris, author of *Men, Love & Birth*, told me that '*when partners go into birth having told themselves it's going to be brutal, even an uncomplicated birth can be shocking*'. Of those who have been to antenatal courses and meetings, many report that these left them underprepared and unclear about their role. Even when birth has gone well, partners may feel shell-shocked by the experience, which can have an impact on their relationship with both their partner and their baby. One study found that 5% of fathers participating reported severe PTSD symptoms after birth (Ayers, Wright and Wells, 2007).

When birth has been traumatic, partners talk about feeling

like 'spectators', excluded during the birth process, powerless to help and unsupported during and after, even when severe and life-threatening complications have been witnessed. New research by Dr Andrew Mayers at Bournemouth University found that fathers feel:

'...marginalised, treated as "secondary partner", were given minimal information about what was happening and what would happen next, were not updated with progress, and received no support for the potential long term impact of witnessing a trauma.'

It's important to note that what partners experience can be very different to the experience of the person who has given birth. This is shown in stories they tell during treatments for trauma, which largely involve retelling the birth story and exploring the meanings that have been made (as described in *How to Heal a Bad Birth*). A partner, experiencing birth as an outsider, without physical sensations informing him or her, and often acting as a conduit between the mother and healthcare professionals, may feel differently about the events witnessed and may also hold distressing information that they felt they needed to keep hidden.

'Every time E caught my eye I'd smile and try and reassure her, but I could see the midwives were getting worried. I felt like I was running from one place to the next, trying to be there for E, getting anything the midwives needed, all while getting more and more concerned that things weren't progressing. No one was taking charge, so I felt I should, but obviously I didn't know what to do.' E.J.

What about same-sex or non-gender-conforming partners?
There is so little research into the experiences of fathers and their birth trauma, that it is perhaps not surprising that there

is no research I have been able to find looking at same-sex partners or non-gender-conforming partners and their experience of birth trauma or the maternity system. However, it is likely that it might be more difficult to access support after birth, due to the lack of resources available and the increased stigma faced by non-heteronormative parents.

'At my first appointment at maternity services at nine weeks pregnant I was handed a set of antenatal notes and asked to fill in my personal information. The form asked for my 'husband's' name and details. When I was taken into my appointment I attempted to explain why I had crossed out that question by saying "The thing is my partner is female" and was told (without the midwife looking up from her notes) "It doesn't matter. Just write his name". I was left a bit confused but got the sense that my sexuality was not welcome.

At an early antenatal appointment I was told that we would be seen in the high-risk clinic, which was news to us. I asked why and was told it was because I had got pregnant through IVF (we hadn't). I explained that we had used at-home artificial insemination and so I couldn't see how that made my pregnancy any more risky than the next person. We were told that once you've been categorised as high-risk you never become not high-risk, so 'that's the route you'll take'. Cue lots of future appointments with people assuming we'd got pregnant a way we hadn't.

My antenatal care was full of low points around the intersection of my pregnancy and my sexuality. Almost every appointment seemed to hold a problem, from disregard of my wife as a 'mother', to using language around the donor that we found emotive and upsetting. A particular low point was the group antenatal class where we were the only same sex couple in a room of 50 couples. The facilitator announced *that she was going to split the room into fathers and mothers for the rest of the day. Panic set in for the two of us, and my partner (who is naturally quite shy and hates to stand out in a crowd) turned to me and said "What will I do?!" She ended up in the group with the men and found it humiliating as it was all about "fathers", and she wasn't acknowledged by the facilitator as being there. We met up at the first break, and made a run for it. We may have missed out on some important information but we were sick of feeling like we didn't belong in the service.' K.*

How does a traumatic birth affect a couple?
As well as directly affecting a partner, through their own witnessing of a traumatic experience, a birth trauma can affect the couple relationship. This, in turn, can have a wider impact on the family dynamic and how able a couple are to co-parent. Even where a partner has not experienced their own traumatic reaction, the impact of the mother or birthing person's continued traumatic stress response can be significant. One qualitative study, which explored the relationships of six couples after a traumatic birth, found that all of the couples felt their relationships had been negatively affected. There are many ways in which a traumatic experience can affect a couple – for example, avoidance of discussing the birth can lead to communication problems.

One area which is certainly not talked about enough postnatally is how much birth can affect a couple's sexual relationship. Most couples find it hard to regain intimacy after birth, and this is compounded by a traumatic birth experience, when a woman or birthing person might be feeling disconnected from their body and understandably afraid of physical intimacy, and a partner may find that sexual activity triggers their own traumatic memories (White, 2007).

Many couples find that speaking to a professional together can help them recover their relationship, and focusing on intimacy rather than sexual contact can be a useful starting point. As well as psychosexual services available on the NHS, there are lots of organisations dedicated to supporting couples after parenthood, such as Relate and the Tavistock Relationships Clinic.

I spoke to Karen Gurney about what can help couples to regain a sexual relationship after a traumatic birth. She said:

'The circumstances we find ourselves in after childbirth are a perfect storm for a drop in desire… not many parents are prepped for the impact having a baby or young kids has on their sex life. It's very normal for sex to fall off the agenda, even without birth trauma. If you also have a birth injury, sex can be painful – and injury to the anal spinchter can really affect body image and self-esteem.

Having a baby or young children is well known to be a time of the lowest sexual satisfaction in a person's life. It's also useful to know that, for most women after a few years with a partner, it's unusual for desire to come 'out of the blue'. Instead desire which is responsive (that needs to be encouraged!) is more common. It's helpful to make some time with your partner, even just a short period, to be physically intimate and just keep your sexual relationship on the agenda. You might want to be naked together, or kiss, or just lie close together talking. Talk to them about any fears you have and how you are feeling. Many people tell me they don't want to draw attention to their fears, in case it turns their partner off, but often it can do the opposite – allowing you both to relax and enjoy sex without the worry of what could go wrong.'

How do I know I'm struggling?
If you're reading this as someone who has witnessed a

traumatic birth (and if you have a partner that fits that bill, do pass this book over to them), you might wonder whether what you are feeling is normal. Well, witnessing a traumatic birth can have a wide-ranging impact, just as it can on the person who has given birth. Partners may also suffer from symptoms of trauma, affecting their mood, their ability to function day to day, the marital relationship and the bond with the baby (which may have an impact on the developing child, too). However, their experience may be further complicated. In previous research, women have talked about feeling resentful and blaming their partner for not 'rescuing' them from their birth, and understandably find it near to impossible to support their partner when they are recovering from their own experience. And partners often feel unjustified in talking about their feelings, feeling instead that they must 'tough it out' (White, 2007). Even if you want and need to talk about your experience, sometimes the support simply isn't available.

If you are reading this and feeling that you would like to speak to someone about your experience, please do check out the 'Seeking Help' section at the back of the book, and all of the information on Healing in Chapter 5 is relevant for both parents as well as others who might feel traumatised.

Trauma in the relationship with the baby

It won't surprise you to learn that a difficult birth can lead to difficulties in the relationship with the baby. Many people feel that they have missed out on the early days of bonding and this sense of loss can permeate their relationship with their baby. The symptoms of PTSD themselves make it difficult to parent – with sleep disturbance exacerbating the sleep deprivation of new parenthood, and the impossibility of avoiding a potential trigger for flashbacks when that trigger is the baby itself.

The symptoms of PTSD and trauma may also manifest in

anxiety about the baby, with symptoms of hypervigilance (an increased sensitivity to threat) being directed to the baby or the baby's health, and heightened anxiety around the baby's wellbeing.

All this makes for difficult reading, I know. All parents want the best for their children and the thought that a bad birth could have a negative impact on your baby too can feel devastating. However, we also know that babies are incredibly adaptable little beings. If you feel that your birth experience is having an impact on your parenting, then please do think about speaking to someone about getting some support.

Most studies exploring bonding have focused on postnatal depression and anxiety rather than traumatic symptoms. Those that have looked at trauma suggest that 'the mother-baby bond [is] also seriously affected' (Ayers et al., 2007). But what we don't yet know is *how* a difficult birth might affect the bond. The Ayers study suggested that a traumatic birth is more likely to lead to an insecure attachment. Attachment relationships are often defined by how sensitive and responsive parents are able to be towards their child, and trauma symptoms may well interfere with this ability to be sensitive. Not only are you preoccupied with your experience, and working hard not to think about it, but you also feel a high level of threat around you which can impact on how you feel, for example when your baby cries. When you've had a difficult birth, you might also feel a sense of resentment towards your child, who can be seen as the cause of that difficulty, making it harder to respond sensitively.

However, it may also be the case that you become overly protective rather than rejecting. When someone goes through a frightening event, during which they felt that lives were at risk, they become hypervigilant to all risk. If you have had the thought during birth that your child might not live, this can colour your experience of that child entirely. Far from being an object of resentment, the baby may come to represent the only positive to come out of the distress – to be protected at all costs. In both events, parenting can become centred around what the baby represents, rather than the baby itself.

> *'Me, well, the psychological trauma haunts me every day and to say I am extremely protective of my son is an understatement.'* J.B.

Added to this is the increased likelihood that you will experience postnatal depression if you are experiencing symptoms of trauma. The influence of postnatal depression on children has been well documented and I won't repeat it here (see *Why Postnatal Depression Matters* by Mia Scotland for a comprehensive view).

Having a traumatic experience of birth can also lead to physical changes that can further impact upon the parenting journey. Physical injury, of course, makes the often physically taxing experience of parenting much more difficult.

The impact on the breastfeeding journey can be a particular source of distress for those who wished to breastfeed. Stress during labour and a long duration of labour have both been shown to affect both onset of lactation (when breastmilk 'comes in') and volume of milk. Many women, feeling a sense of failure after their traumatic birth experience, feel additional pressure to 'succeed' at breastfeeding, creating additional anxiety and feelings of shame. The research on breastfeeding difficulties reflects many of the same themes as we see in birth trauma research – the expectation that it will be 'natural' and the shock and feelings of guilt when it turns out not to be this way. Beck, Driscoll and Watson (2013) suggest that women who have experienced traumatic childbirth should be offered intensive one-to-one support for breastfeeding if desired.

'As it happened, I couldn't face caring for [my son] at all. He was looked after by the midwife because I didn't even want to look at him. Doctors advised me not to breastfeed – after all, I could hardly keep myself going, let alone myself and a baby. The chance to build a connection was taken away from me because I had to spend so much time looking after myself.' J.P.

The impact on the relationship with the baby, of course, is not restricted to the early days of parenting. Birthdays – representing the anniversary of the traumatic experience – can reignite feelings of distress and trauma. This can be doubly distressing as parents are aware that they don't want the traumatic birth to overshadow their feelings about their child. The far-reaching impact of a difficult childbirth in this way really demonstrates why it is so very important that we improve the experiences of parents during birth.

What is most remarkable is that parents who have been through a traumatic birth experience somehow manage to set aside the very distressing symptoms of trauma in order to meet the needs of their children, sometimes at tremendous cost to themselves. While it is very hard reading about the potential impact on a baby, I would urge you to read the next chapter about healing from a difficult birth and have a look at the 'Seeking Help' section. Resolving your own feelings about a traumatic birth can have an enormously positive influence on your relationships – and it's never too late.

Trauma in medical staff

Although the 'second victim' concept was coined in reference to medical professionals, we rarely consider the feelings of doctors and midwives when dealing with difficult births. There seems to be an expectation that, because it is their job, they won't experience vicarious trauma. However, there is increasing awareness that health professionals are not only emotionally

The Second Victim

affected, but that this also impacts upon their care.

There is very little research in this area, although in one survey 15% of Swedish obstetricians and midwives reported PTSD symptoms after their 'worst obstetric event' (Wahlberg et al., 2017), and another study on labour and delivery nurses found that 35% of this sample reported moderate to severe levels of secondary traumatic stress (Beck and Gable, 2012). As we have learned in previous chapters, the role of interpersonal care is also important here. Midwives who feel they have witnessed poor care are likely to experience more severe post-traumatic stress than where birth trauma hasn't involved an interpersonal element (Leinweber et al., 2017).

> Dr Sally Pezaro, academic midwife
>
> *'As a midwife, I joined the profession to do great things. Indeed, research shows that this is the case for the majority of midwives. No one joins the profession to make mistakes or do bad things. Yet, as we navigate through our career journeys, some are praised only for "going above and beyond".*
>
> *Furthermore, phrases are bandied about such as "put the patient first", but where does that leave the midwife? Second? Third? Fourth? Childbearing should be a positive experience for all: for me that means the midwife too.*
>
> *Yet all too often, the midwife, in his/her pursuit to "do great things", is often left in psychological distress with the idea that this is because they are lacking in "resilience". It is in fact a complex combination of organisational, individual and sociocultural factors which actually come together and create the hostile environment in which some midwives are unable to remain psychologically safe. Put it this way, if a flower fails to bloom, you don't fix the flower, you look to fix its environment, right?*

Where healthcare staff experience work-related psychological distress, rates of medical error, infection and morbidity increase. Furthermore, those affected can endure challenging behavioural and physical symptoms of ill health. Personally, I suffered greatly with work-related psychological distress while in clinical practice. I was left professionally broken and needing to rebuild both myself and my professional identity. As such, I began PhD research to develop an online intervention designed to support midwives in work-related psychological distress and increase people's awareness of work-related psychological distress in healthcare.

Findings from our latest research reveal that childbearing women are currently seeing midwives cry, display poor workplace behaviours, become emotional and seek support from them and their families. This is not conducive to a positive experience for anyone in maternity services. Ultimately, the wellbeing of maternity staff can be directly linked to the safety and quality of maternity care. Consequently, it behoves all of society to invest in the wellbeing of midwives.

My ongoing vision for the future is to work in partnership with maternity services, patients and the public to achieve excellence in maternity care. Yet this vision may only be realised once maternity service improvement strategies appreciate an equal focus upon effective midwifery workplace support.'

The recent book *This is Going to Hurt* by Adam Kay, about his experience as a junior doctor on a maternity ward, reveals a great deal about the culture in which obstetricians are expected to work and how little compassion is given to staff when dealing with distressing situations. In the final chapters of the book, Kay describes a number of highly difficult events, frequently working in one emergency situation after another having not eaten or slept for hours. The death of a mother and baby, which led to his leaving medicine, seems almost inevitable in these circumstances – where early warning signs could not possibly be noticed.

Research has focused largely on the way that such 'adverse events' are dealt with within an organisational culture, where they are often responded to in a punitive and blaming rather than supportive manner, making it less likely that staff will disclose errors. For doctors, there is evidence that committing an error can lead to depression, burnout, anxiety, shame and guilt. Dr Sally Pezaro's work with midwives suggests that they too are dealing with stress, not only from their role supporting women, but also from doing so in an environment which places coping and sacrifice on a pedestal, leading them to keep working despite their distress. It is clear that such an emotional impact will affect a professional's ability to care. A Royal College of Physicians (2015) report found a 'clear correlation between staff health and the quality of patient care'. Dr Pezaro's research highlights how working under such pressure leads to a reduced ability to care, and 'compassion fatigue'. Kay, in his book, describes how risk averse his experiences made him, saying 'I couldn't risk anything bad ever happening again.... I knew women were having unnecessary caesareans... but if it meant everyone got out of there alive it was worth it'.

I spoke to Caroline Wright, obstetrician and gynaecologist, about her experience of birth trauma. Please read with caution, as this contains a story about bereavement and is upsetting to read.

Dr Caroline Wright, obstetrician and gynaecologist

'The intense working environment of our speciality, plus witnessing birth trauma, makes a heavy mental load for obstetricians. A shocking 89% of obstetric trainees reported feeling low in mood or anxious in a speciality survey, and the attrition rate for trainees is around 30%. Trauma among staff may well be a contributing factor.

A day I particularly remember as traumatic was as a junior registrar years ago. I came in early to start my weekend shift and immediately was needed in theatre. A woman in labour, the baby was extremely premature (25 weeks). A decision had been taken with the couple to perform a caesarean as a last resort. The operation became complicated and the baby was very difficult to deliver. Though I was only assisting the operation, it was my smaller hands that eventually managed to guide the baby out. As I cupped the tiny infant in my hands, I knew there was little hope. The parents, of course, were extremely distressed and throughout the operation I heard their heartbreaking sobs. I remember crying in the toilets afterwards, the whole experience had been so horrific. It was only 8:30am… I had 12 more hours to get through, antenatal and postnatal patients to see and a full labour ward of women to look after. I had to pull myself together and deal with the busy day, lots of healthy babies born, but the trauma of the first delivery was still with me. I was so glad to see my colleague come to take over at 8pm. It was still busy, so she went to theatre for me, leaving me to see just one more patient. Sadly, as I ran the scanner over the woman's 38-week tummy… I found no heartbeat. Breaking the bad news was so hard.

Later at home I broke down, intense images from the day flashing through my brain that stay with me even now.

Nobody asked if I was ok.

Learning about how trauma affects staff is so important. We can do our jobs better when we support each other.'

Although increased funding has gone into maternity services, they are still under extreme pressure. The WHELM study, commissioned by the Royal College of Midwives and published this year, found a workforce in crisis. Midwives leave the profession quickly, and more than a third of those who responded were moderately to severely depressed, anxious and stressed and 83% were suffering from burnout. There is a similar story for obstetricians. The 2017 Royal College of Obstetricians and Gynaecologists Workforce Report painted a picture of a workforce thinking of or actively leaving, facing increasing staffing gaps and increased work pressure.

Many healthcare professionals also come to the profession with their own birth stories – those from their own births, from family members and friends, and their own ideas about what birth might look like. In many ways, their own experiences can shape their practice, for good and bad. Carl Jung talked about 'the wounded healer' – describing how many people become 'healers' (in his case, a psychotherapist) because of their own 'wounds'. In this way, we heal ourselves through healing others. Many of those who enter the maternity profession may do so both to heal their own birth traumas and to prevent a re-enactment of the traumatic stories they have been told. Of course, when the maternity system puts them in a position where they feel they are contributing to trauma, this can then be doubly distressing.

Here, specialist mental health midwife Hannah Horne talks about how her birth experience has influenced her own practice:

'Being a midwife who experienced birth trauma as a mother has professionally given me a unique experience. I was aware on my return to work that my birth experience had the potential to affect my practice as a midwife, because it had such an

impact on me. I was mindful that this had the potential to be positive or negative; I did not want my experience to negatively impact any of the women in my care. I felt the fact that I was able to recognise this as a possibility meant that it was highly unlikely to, but I was definitely aware of this. When I returned to work I felt like I was viewing the whole process of birth differently. Prior to becoming a mother myself I was in awe of birth and motherhood, I firmly believed in physiological birth and supported women through that process and supported them if any medical interventions were required. I had supported women to examine their choices around birth and counselled them through making choices that weren't within guidelines and involved other professionals as required. When I returned to work I saw that women tend to have a lot of choice around low-risk and physiological birth, but when birth becomes high-risk or requiring medical interventions then care can be less individualised and could lack a human element. While I had always been aware of this and tried to bring low-risk elements of care to higher-risk settings, when I returned to work following my birth experience it was as if this reality was staring me in the face. I was less likely to wait until women requested certain aspects of care such as skin-to-skin in theatre and I actively offered and encouraged it. I made small changes by making sure parents saw their baby as it was born by C-section and bringing the scales to the parents rather than weighing the baby on the other side of the theatre where the scales were kept for convenience. While some of these small changes in practice weren't always possible, I would promote them and carry them out as much as possible. Now with more hospitals offering family-centred or 'natural' c-sections, high-risk birth experiences are changing for the better, which will hopefully help to reduce rates of birth trauma, as that element of control can be really important in reducing trauma or promoting recovery from trauma.

Another element of my practice that has benefited from my experience is that I can use it to really empathise with women when they are struggling with a difficult birth experience, a difficult motherhood experience or if they are having difficulties with their mental health. Through my experience, educating myself on birth trauma and accessing training days, I really understand how birth trauma can happen and how it can manifest in women's physical and mental health. This allows me to educate women on what birth trauma is and how that can make them feel. It doesn't take the trauma away, but by understanding what is happening in their body and mind it becomes less frightening. I can support them through their mental health difficulties and trauma symptoms because I can speak from my experience and from the heart. I can make suggestions for how they can soothe their hyperalert systems and encourage mindfulness and relaxation. I don't discuss details of my own birth experience, but will tell women in my care that I had a traumatic birth and that I got better and that is very reassuring and gives them hope that they too will recover. I also use my own experience in training midwives and other professionals. When I look back at my traumatic birth experience I value it, not only because it brought me my son and made me a mother, despite the fact that it was difficult to experience and recover from, but also because it gave me such an insight into the vulnerability women experience through their journey through pregnancy, labour, birth and early motherhood. With my knowledge as an experienced midwife I walked into pregnancy with my eyes wide open. Had my pregnancy, birth and early motherhood period been straightforward I would have had a lovely, positive experience, but I might not have known how vulnerable some woman can feel throughout this process. Having experienced vulnerability around birth trauma and motherhood I can understand the vulnerability of the women in my care more fully and comprehend their anxiety, their concern and issues with their mental health more effectively. It is as if I am walking alongside them, viewing maternity services from their point of view. It allows me to understand and advocate for them more effectively. I can help them to understand their own emotions, I can help them to voice them, I can support them to make decisions regarding their care and I can support them in conversations with other professionals to ensure their needs are met. I am a firm believer in everything happening for a reason; I believe the birth I experienced and the aftermath allowed me to have a service-user experience of the psychological journey through pregnancy, birth and adjustment to motherhood, with the professional knowledge of a midwife. I can use my experience to improve care for women and to work alongside other professionals to improve emotional care within maternity services as a whole.'

Without adequate support for the emotional consequences of traumatic births for staff as well as patients, there is a danger that services themselves can become traumatised – hypervigilant to risk, avoidant of reflecting on difficult events and finding it impossible to see any potential positives in the birth process. This is something we are actively trying to change with Make Birth Better – encouraging services to recognise that their reactive way of working may be increasing the risk of trauma for both parents and staff.

If you are reading this as a professional, the information on healing is also relevant to you. You may also wish to get involved with our Make Birth Better campaign.

Trauma in society

In modern UK society in 2018, we have a very mixed view of birth. On the one hand, there is the prevailing medical model, viewing birth as a medical event which carries risk. On the other there is the natural birth movement, which portrays birth as a physiological event which can bring empowerment. While conversations about birth are often passionate and heartfelt, such a dichotomy can itself be seen as a traumatic reaction – in which urgency and adrenaline overpower the capacity for reflection.

This is not surprising given the way that birth is often portrayed in the media, as a dramatic experience, which takes place in burnt-out maternity services. In parallel, there remains a reluctance to talk openly about birth. It becomes a secretive experience, with any problems quickly dismissed with a 'well, a healthy baby is all that matters'. This reflects a lack of understanding of how life-changing birth can be – both positively and negatively.

Our natural response to anxiety is often to try and assert more control in order to take away fear-provoking uncertainty. But here is the trouble with birth – it is in its very nature unpredictable. And, while there are ways in which it can be made more predictable, as a society it seems hard to live with the unsettling fact that birth can be both positive and harrowing, and sometimes both in the same birth.

Just as we treat individual trauma by hearing stories and listening to interpretations, we can do the same with services. By hearing from and listening to all the people involved in birth and understanding how they respond to difficult and traumatic situations, we can start to heal.

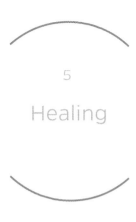

5

Healing

There are now many techniques available to those who wish to heal after a traumatic birth experience, whether this is to help recover from symptoms of PTSD or more general symptoms of trauma or perinatal distress. Many of these are available on the NHS, although depending on the area in which you live you may need to join a waiting list. You may also wish to speak to a voluntary sector organisation or independent practitioner about what they can offer. There are many listed on the Make Birth Better map, and you are also welcome to add services or practitioners you are aware of on to this map if they are not listed.

The first step to healing, however, is recognising that your birth was not the experience that you wanted, and that it was not your fault that things did not go the way you'd hoped. There is such a pressure on individuals to 'succeed' at birth, that a difficult birth ends up as a personal 'failure'. We don't question the stories that tell us that birth can be magical if only we try hard enough. Instead we question ourselves and hide our distress because of the shame this causes.

When birth is traumatic, this can be for a variety of reasons (as outlined in Chapter 2), but none of these reasons are your fault. Sometimes they are the fault of medical professionals, sometimes they are the fault of the wider medical system, sometimes they are even the fault of other circumstances within society or your life. You are not responsible for having a bad birth.

Once we can acknowledge that birth hasn't gone well, and that the way we are feeling is not part of the normal process of birth recovery, then we have made the first step towards healing. Instead of blaming ourselves, we can start to be kind to ourselves and look for the support that can help us reconnect with our bodies and minds. And instead of blaming ourselves, we can also start to question whether there are others who should be held accountable.

There are many different ways you can treat symptoms of trauma. You may find that, over time, you use a combination of different techniques as you move towards recovering.

Becoming safe again

Most of the treatments which are recommended for symptoms of trauma involve exploring the traumatic memory in some way and integrating it into the normal long-term memory store.

However, across all fields there is a general understanding that this can only be done in the context of *safety*. Traumatic events challenge our understanding that we are safe, putting our bodies into 'survival mode'. Symptoms of trauma repeatedly tell our bodies and minds that we are not safe. So the key to recovery is to learn that you and those around you are now safe again.

Before beginning any memory-focused treatment, you will be encouraged to learn how to get yourself into that place of safety. For some this may involve body techniques such as breathing, or you might visualise a 'safe place'. You can practise these yourself to target those physiological symptoms of trauma. For some people, memory-focused treatments may feel too difficult and you might choose to only practice grounding techniques to help you manage your own symptoms.

What is grounding?

When we are in our 'fight or flight' response, our whole body feels that we are under threat. Our prefrontal cortex goes offline and our actions are taken over by the amygdala, our alarm system. We are entirely in survival mode, our bodies full of adrenaline. When we have PTSD, or traumatic symptoms, we can exist in this place for long periods of time. This is why we might find it difficult to concentrate, respond to things impulsively, forget things and feel irritated. We are in a state of emergency all the time.

Grounding can really help us let our bodies know that we are safe. Here are a couple of techniques that can help. Do consider sharing them with the people around you too – they may find them useful if they have some symptoms of trauma themselves, or they can remind you of these techniques when needed.

Breathing

When we are in our fight or flight mode, our sympathetic nervous system is working to get us to a place of safety. If we are, in fact, safe, we need to 'switch on' our parasympathetic nervous system, otherwise known as the 'rest and digest' system. The quickest way of doing this is by focusing on the out-breath.

Take a deep breath in through your nose and a longer, slower breath out through your mouth. Keep doing this, with your out-breath always longer. This signals to the body that you are safe and it is ok to rest. (Notice that the opposite will happen if you take short, sharp inward breaths which pump oxygen to your limbs and get you ready for action!).

You might want to make that out breath audible, or you might want to sigh it out, or even roar it out! There is a yoga breath called 'Lion's Roar' which can feel very grounding, during which you stick your tongue out and open your mouth wide and gently 'roar' out your out-breath. Experiment and see what feels most comfortable for you.

Use your senses

Using your five senses can quickly take you out of your emergency mode, reminding you that you are safe and bringing you into the present and out of that traumatic experience. One way of doing this is by consciously looking for one thing you can see, one thing you can hear, one thing you can smell, one thing you can taste and one thing you can touch. You can again experiment with this, perhaps looking for all of the triangles you can see in the room, or all of the yellow objects – whatever you feel is a useful tool for you to use. This can be especially helpful when you are starting to feel lost in a traumatic memory, or if a trigger (such as the smell of disinfectant) has brought on a flashback.

The importance of sleep

Some research has demonstrated a link between poor sleep and symptoms of PTSD. We know from a huge body of research into sleep that poor sleep can affect our mood, behaviour and physical health in a range of different ways. Alleviating any symptoms of insomnia can really help to reduce trauma symptoms.

A quick lesson on sleep hygiene

Many of us have really terrible sleep habits! We stay up late and get up too early, often interrupted in the night by small children. We take our phones to bed, or watch TV until we fall asleep. We lie in on the weekends. All of these things interrupt our circadian rhythms and affect the quality of our sleep. Here are five things to try to improve your sleep:

1. Try and go to bed at the same time each night, and wake up at the same time. This can be very difficult with small children, but try and time your bedtime in line with their wake time.
2. Keep your bedroom pitch black, and cool.
3. Turn off all screens at least an hour before bed. Leave them in another room to reduce temptation to check.
4. Just as you do with your children, have a regular wind-down routine. A bath with magnesium salts, a wind-down meditation, some stretching – anything to signal to your body that you are getting ready for sleep.
5. If you continue to have trouble sleeping, please speak to your GP.

Psychological treatments

In the UK, within the NHS we have the National Institute for Health and Care Excellence (NICE) guidelines, which outline the recommended treatments for all mental and physical health problems. You can read through these yourself on the NICE website if you would like to see what you should be entitled to in any aspect of your healthcare.

At present, the advice for those who have experienced a traumatic birth is the same as for general PTSD symptoms.

The recommended advice for PTSD is that it would usually be recognised at a primary care level – by your GP or another healthcare professional such as a midwife. Any professional you come into contact with should be aware of the symptoms of PTSD, be flexible about how a service is offered, make sure you can access those services, offer a choice of therapist and think about your whole family and how they might also be affected by the traumatic birth (this is in line with the most recent 2018 NICE guidance).

There is an argument that the NICE guidelines rely heavily on Randomised Controlled Trials (RCTs), and many clinicians have called for the use of other methods of evaluating effective therapies to allow for a broader and more innovative approach to treatments. At present, the recommended treatment for PTSD is either a course of Trauma Focused Cognitive Behavioural Therapy (TF-CBT), or Eye Movement Desensitisation and Reprocessing (EMDR) treatment, as these are the two treatments with the strongest evidence base. Both of these therapies should be available to you within your local talking therapies service. Although not explicitly created for those affected by traumatic symptoms after birth, researchers have suggested that they are effective, although they also call for further research in this area.

It is worth noting that single sessions of therapy or debriefing focusing on 'reliving' the traumatic event *are not recommended* for anyone experiencing PTSD, whether birth-related or not. This is because, without an opportunity to process the traumatic memory, going over it in this way can be re-traumatising. At the very least, it is not likely to feel helpful. Despite this, the current NHS system of offering debriefing sessions after birth or asking patients to go through a triage assessment to access help can often lead to multiple occasions of having to go over (and over) the traumatic event. Debriefing sessions are also often offered in the hospital in which you were traumatised – something which is advised against in the NICE guidance. If you find that this is happening to you, it is worth bearing in mind that you are entitled to withhold the details of your traumatic experience until you are with a clinician who is able to devote the appropriate time and attention to your story, and you are able to request a session in a different location (in accordance with the NICE guidance).

While a small percentage of women (around 4%) might meet the criteria for PTSD, there is also a far greater number of people – women and birthing people, their partners, and those around them including family members and healthcare professionals – who may be affected by some post-traumatic stress symptoms, or feel a more general sense of perinatal distress (in which a difficult birth is one of many other factors). For those with diagnosable PTSD, treatments other than those recommended by the NICE guidelines would not be advised, as there is a potential to worsen the symptoms of trauma. For those who have some symptoms or a more general sense of distress, there are other treatments and techniques available which do not yet have an evidence base to support their use but may still be extremely helpful. If you are considering seeking support, I would urge you to research both testimonials and criticisms of the approach you are looking into. If you have a history of traumatic experiences, any practice which emphasises techniques such as grounding can be helpful – but any technique which dives into memories can be deeply distressing. If you feel that any of your symptoms are worsening, please share that with whoever is conducting the treatment or technique with you, and if necessary speak to your GP. Birth and the world around birth has become a huge industry in recent years and there are many well-meaning and wonderful people who wish to help those who have been through a difficult experience – but there is also the capacity to do harm. Choose a practitioner carefully and, if you don't feel that you are being helped, don't be afraid to seek an alternative. Within the NHS, there are complaints procedures you can follow (outlined below).

With that slightly alarming paragraph out of the way, I'd also like to say that treatments for PTSD and trauma symptoms can be extremely effective, with symptoms often being alleviated rapidly. Once you find the right person or the right tool to suit you, you may be amazed at how quickly the burden of trauma can be lifted.

The reality of the NHS in 2019

While treatments should be widely available on the NHS I hear from more and more people who tell me they have found it next to impossible to get a referral to a trauma specialist or a perinatal specialist. Or, in fact, to get a referral to anyone at all.

The majority of people needing support following a traumatic birth will not meet the diagnostic criteria necessary to warrant a referral to secondary care mental health services such as perinatal mental health teams or trauma-specific services (although some teams choose to see those who don't meet thresholds in order to fill this gap).

Over the past 10 years, the combination of the Improving Access to Psychological Therapies (IAPT) service (ostensibly to widen access to therapy by providing CBT to those with mild to moderate mental health problems) and the cuts to the NHS because of austerity policies have resulted in the decline of psychology as a profession within primary care mental health services. In many talking therapies services there is little to no perinatal specialist training or supervision, and psychologists are leaving (or feeling pushed out of) the NHS. A recent wellbeing survey of psychological practitioners found that many are concerned about the safety and effectiveness of mental health services within the NHS, with the loss of more highly qualified members of staff leading to a lack of confidence in many teams. The remaining workforce within talking therapies report high staff turnover and high levels of burnout. One psychological wellbeing practitioner (a junior member of staff offering brief CBT), who wanted to remain anonymous, told me:

'IAPT continues to attempt to meet the NHS England Guidelines following particular recommendations of the Five-Year Forward Plan to increase support for women in the perinatal period. New timeline recommendations have been brought in, namely perinatal patients to be assessed within two weeks and into treatment within four weeks. Needless to say, services are struggling to meet those deadlines. This is leading to patients being placed with any clinician, whether or not they are experienced or trained in providing perinatal care.

That is not to say that these guidelines are not appropriate – they are absolutely the standards of care we should be providing. However, they are unrealistic without extra resources and only serve to stretch already limited resources even further.

I have been tasked (as a trainee as well as when qualified as a PWP) to provide therapy for clients with complex mental health difficulties, trauma, historical sexual abuse, previous birth trauma… This has been detrimental to their wellbeing – as not one of those clients has reached 'clinical recovery' on discharge. They are offered four 30-minute sessions, and leave feeling they are not better and cannot get better.

We are mostly focused on women who are due to or have given birth who are also experiencing a mental health difficulty. What we often fail to consider as well, is women who have lost children in pregnancy or birth, individuals in same-sex relationships who are not classed as 'perinatal' if they are not carrying their child, women who are losing

*children through IVF, fathers who are struggling with
bonding or their own mental health difficulties. There is a
whole spectrum of people whom childbirth affects and they
are not being supported.*

    *It is not that therapists are not trying their hardest, because
they really are. PWP's are the most hardworking individuals
I have ever come across – often seeing upwards of 35 patients
per week and managing highly complex clients. However, as
a 25-year-old with no children and no experience of perinatal
mental healthcare I hold my hands up to say I do not have the
skills or experience to help these women. In having tried to, I
fear I am doing more harm than good.'*

Why am I telling you this? At present, there is a widening
disparity between NHS guidance (such as the Five Year
Forward Plan, the IAPT Positive Practice Perinatal
Guidance and the Maternity Transformation plan), which
all emphasise the need for quick and effective specialist
perinatal mental health care and the reality of many NHS
services. Many people contact me having been to speak
to their GP or another healthcare professional and, upon
finding that there is no service available to them, assume that
they have to struggle on in silence. That their problem can't
be that bad, perhaps it's normal, and they are not entitled to
support. Or, they are referred for six sessions of CBT and
leave feeling that their problems are not solvable.

The NICE guidelines state (among many other things)
that, for people who have PTSD, different treatment choices
should be offered in line with their preferences, family
members should also be held in mind, that professionals
should be aware of the barriers to accessing treatment
for people with these symptoms, that treatment should
be given by competent individuals who have appropriate
supervision, and that flexibility over treatment duration

and location should be offered.

Services around the UK are struggling to meet national NHS guidelines. If this has happened to you, please complain to your local NHS commissioner or speak to the Patient Advice and Liaison Service (PALS). You can find out how to do this on the NHS England website ('How do I feedback or make a complaint about an NHS service').

The 2013 MIND *We still need to talk* report found that 1 in 10 people waited for over a year to receive therapeutic intervention, 58% were not offered choice in the therapy they received and 11% of respondents had paid for therapy outside the NHS. The report states:

> 'For the Government to achieve its own parity of esteem duty, urgent action is needed to continue to expand and improve psychological therapy provision in the UK. It is not enough to pledge equality for people with mental health problems when in reality local services are dealing with an ever increasing demand for psychological therapies.'

The two psychological treatments most commonly used by the NHS and trauma-focused psychological specialists are both focused on targeting the traumatic memory. They allow the exploration of the memory of the trauma and the meanings attributed to it, and then work to reintegrate the memory within the long-term memory system. Based on the models described in Chapter 2, this enables the 'fight or flight' element of the memory to dissipate. In this way, the traumatic experience becomes a memory much like any other – accessed as an experience, but without the depth of emotional response that comes with a traumatic memory. While TF-CBT and EMDR on the surface look like quite different treatments, they have been found to be equally successful for the treatment of PTSD.

While these treatments are effective for those struggling

with symptoms of trauma after birth, so far little research has been done looking at which psychological treatments are most effective specifically for parents. Clinical psychologist Kirstie McKenzie-McHarg has suggested that anyone working in this area should be aware that there may need to be special consideration given to the experience of women or birthing people and their partners. While others suffering from symptoms of PTSD after a traumatic event will usually have the experience of their trauma acknowledged by those around them, after birth we have the unique experience that we are expected to be happy and grateful. This can really add to the traumatic experience, in that we don't feel able to express it. The baby itself can act as a reminder of the trauma, so there is a difficulty in moving past the trauma, which doesn't exist for other traumatic experiences. Finally, because of the stigma around feeling that we have 'failed' at birth (or 'failed' to protect our partner from a difficult birth), alongside thoughts about the baby we may feel ashamed of, it is especially important that the clinical setting feels like a safe space for both the parent and the baby.

Trauma-focused CBT

Based on the Ehlers and Clark model described in Chapter 1, trauma-focused CBT allows us to work through all of the different factors which might be keeping the trauma memory alive. This will usually include a combination of different approaches, such as learning techniques, like grounding strategies, to ensure that we can manage the physical symptoms of trauma and calm down the threat response that can be triggered by the memory of the trauma. Often the birth story is talked through in detail, and may be written about to identify the parts which seem most upsetting, and the negative meaning attributed at these times (called 'hotspots'). These are then talked through in detail and alternative meanings are constructed together. Going through the birth story with these new, often kinder, meanings can help to integrate the traumatic memory into the normal autobiographical memory, taking away the strong emotional reaction it creates.

You may also go through other techniques such as: exposure to the place in which the trauma took place (such as visiting the labour ward using grounding techniques to bring down the 'it's an emergency' threat response), identifying particular triggers and learning to manage these situations by highlighting the difference between the time of the event and what is happening in the present, or using imagery to strongly integrate a feeling of safety. You might also go through what seemingly insignificant things you may be doing day to day which could be adding to symptoms of trauma (for example, avoiding healthcare professionals if you feel that seeing a professional may trigger traumatic memories).

Many TF-CBT models also allow us to process any shame we hold alongside the traumatic experience. This seems to be particularly pertinent when we have experienced a traumatic birth. Newer 'third wave' cognitive behavioural models have targeted that experience of shame, by introducing a kinder and more compassionate meaning to the traumatic memory.

In my work, I have tended to lean towards a TF-CBT model (which is why it is described in such detail here!). Here is one exercise you might find helpful (you can do this exercise if you feel that you have been traumatised by witnessing, being involved in or hearing about a traumatic birth too).

Telling your story

If you feel that you have been affected by your birth experience or a birth experience you witnessed, you may wish to write out your memory of the birth and follow these steps. However, if you have a history of trauma before birth, or you are living in a situation which continues to leave you feeling traumatised, or you have severe symptoms of PTSD, then I would not recommend that you do this. Instead, please seek help from a mental health professional who will do this work alongside you, ensuring that you are kept safe throughout.

If you feel that you have support around you and feel that you have the internal resources to manage any difficult feelings, then you may wish to write out your own birth story. You can also ask your birth partner or your partner who gave birth to write their version of events. If you, or they, notice that you are feeling very distressed, or that writing it out triggers a flashback in which you feel that you are 'back there', please use the grounding techniques and seek some support.

The purpose of this exercise is to create a fluid narrative of the birth experience, draw out some of the meanings you attributed to events during the birth, to process some of the emotions related to them, and to file away that memory again with your other long-term memories, taking away some of that strong emotional resonance.

Write out the birth story as fully as you possibly can, paying attention to details and also to how you feel while writing. Think about what it meant to you, what you feel most affected by now and the reason for this. The meaning you have attributed to particular events may surprise you: for example, it may not be that you are angry that you had an emergency c-section when you had planned a home birth – but that you feel a sense of shame that you 'failed' to have the birth you wanted. It may not be that you are angry about the rude remark made to you by a midwife, but that you felt sidelined as a birth partner throughout the experience. It may not be that you are distressed at the difficult physical experience you had, but felt violated by an internal examination. As a professional, it may not be that you were involved in a traumatic experience, but that this left you feeling helpless.

Think about what those situations or experiences meant to you – about you as a person, about the world around you, about birth, about people. Are you making any judgements on yourself or those around you? How did you feel at the time? Were you scared? Angry? Out of control? What did you think was going to happen? Often you'll know that you've hit upon the 'true' meaning because you'll feel a big lump in your throat or the tears will flow. Write it all down – it all counts.

When you've written everything down, have a read through everything again. If your birth partner or your partner who gave birth has written their version of events, you can read through each other's and talk it through together. If you are not doing this with a partner, you might want to find someone you trust to be kind to talk through your birth story with.

With all the knowledge you have now about how things turned out – how you are now, how your baby is now, why certain decisions were made – tell your story again. Pick up on those parts that made your heart hurt and think about new ways of interpreting them or ask your birth partner or someone else to help you think of other interpretations. Maybe 'I failed' turns into 'I didn't have the support I needed'. Or 'They violated me' becomes 'They needed to act quickly and couldn't consider my feelings'. Or 'I didn't do enough' starts to look like 'I did the best I could'. Or 'I could have lost my baby' is replaced with 'I now know my baby is healthy and safe'. Do this as many times as you need to, and rewrite it if you want with the new appraisals that you've made. What you're doing is pulling that information away from the emergency system and using your long-term memory systems to file it away. So it can join all the other times you had contact with medics, the times you coped well in times of stress, and the history of your life as a parent so far.

You may find, in doing this exercise, that you become angry

at the way you were treated during your birth, or there may be examples of negligence. If this is the case, please see the section later in this chapter on making a complaint.

What does it feel like to have CBT?
I asked Make Birth Better lived experience contributor Jo Page to tell me about her experience of CBT. As mentioned earlier in the chapter, sometimes different therapies will be beneficial at different times – and Jo's experience really exemplifies how important it is to find a therapist that fits with you:

'I have had three blocks of face-to-face CBT in the last 23 years since my birth trauma, and one block of telephone CBT too. The first block of face-to-face was based around a whiteboard, lots of writing and drawing speech bubbles and me using the board too. I will be totally honest: my trauma was that bad and my physical injury also causing such problems that I didn't see how this could help me. At that time, I needed something more compassionate – not having to participate in such physical activities in the session.

My second face-to-face block was a trial, mixing the CBT with physical exercise. This was good but not on the NHS and so expensive. It really helped me to do both – I had homework and exercises to do.

The telephone CBT I really found hard to get into, this wasn't for me. The therapist was nice but her ways of helping me cope with my fears of dying were just not helpful.

The last CBT I had was the best for me. It was a 10-week block with an older lady who was very good at her job! I went there in a state, with some very upsetting thoughts. At the end I was a different person. We had no whiteboard, she let me talk and each session asked me what I wanted to discuss that week and at the end checked I had got the answers I needed.

I had homework each session, very focused on my goals. For example, I knew I needed to get my physical birth injuries looked at but was so nervous about seeing a consultant. She talked me through how to use breathing to keep calm, and my thoughts about going. I was in charge of all of the sessions. She saved me.'

I also spoke to Becky, whose birth was traumatic because it triggered memories of her previous experiences of abuse:

'One of the first things I was taught was breathing exercises. I had to put my hand on my stomach and breathe in and out – breathing out for longer than breathing in. I'd already used this method to help calm myself down before, but it was useful to remember how powerful breathing can be.

One time when I got quite distressed in a session, my therapist just said 'let's look at all the things in the room that are blue'. And then we listed them. This helped me calm down in other situations, by just noticing what was around me.

My therapist told me to close my eyes and think of going to a place where I felt safe, peaceful and calm. I imagined going to my grandma and grandad's garden when I was younger. I'd sit on the bench under the tree and look at what was around me. The season, the smells, the time of day, the weather, even imagining my grandma and grandad being there.

I think the other exercises were her just talking me through what had happened and changing my thoughts around that. Challenging why I was thinking certain things. For example, I thought I wasn't a good mum, so she had me tell her what I thought a good mum was, tell her what I thought a bad mum was, and talk about examples of good and bad mums I knew in my life and where I was on that scale.

I found that going through the process of CBT was fairly difficult during some of the sessions, because it brought up very strong past emotions. It was full on at times, but I left each session feeling good. The process helped me to reorganise my feelings and get rid of the guilt I was feeling. It really made me feel so much better about myself and about the birth experience I had, and why it went how it did.'

EMDR*

EMDR therapy brings together a number of different psychotherapies into one highly effective treatment. Although very different from CBT, it works in a similar way by allowing the traumatic memories to be integrated into the long-term memory system. In this way, useful and positive information is held on to, while the more negative and highly emotional aspects of the memory take on less influence.

EMDR follows a strict protocol, with eight phases of treatment. It is crucial that each phase is followed:

1. History taking and planning for therapy

The therapist will conduct a detailed assessment, asking about your personal history and creating a plan for the therapy. This will include identifying particular targets for the EMDR treatment – such as the traumatic event, but also things that are happening in the present which might be causing you distress, and anything that it would be helpful for you to learn about during therapy.

2. Preparation

The therapist will explain how EMDR works and teach a number of techniques to help you deal with any difficult feelings that emerge during the EMDR phase of the treatment. These might include grounding techniques, identifying a 'safe place' and also building resources to support you during your therapy.

---

* With thanks to Helen Tudor, clinical psychologist.

3. Assessment

You will identify a particular image or scene which you strongly relate to the traumatic memory, and the negative thought or meaning that you associate with it. You'll also identify any physical or emotional sensations you attach to the event. You will then think of a more positive appraisal you would like to associate with the experience.

4. Desensitization

The therapist will use a tool to create a 'dual awareness', which will allow you to process the memory while also attending to something else such as a finger movement, tapping or tones. This enables the traumatic memory to be processed.

5. Installation

The new, more positive belief is integrated (this must be something believable, such as 'now I am safe' and often refers to yourself in some way). You'll also identify any physical or emotional sensations you associate with the memory, and the level of distress the memory causes you. You will then think of a more positive appraisal you would like to associate with the experience.

6. Body scan

You are encouraged to scan your body for any signs of tension, which are then targeted for further reprocessing. This is because trauma can be held in the body and may not always be accessible in a narrative, so in this way all of the symptoms of trauma are targeted.

7. Closure

You are encouraged to use calming techniques to ensure that you leave every session feeling grounded. The therapist may also ask you about how you found the experience of processing, and let you know about anything you might expect between sessions as processing continues (such as dreams, new insights or memories being raised).

8. Re-evaluation

At the beginning of each session, the therapist will check to see how positive beliefs are being strengthened, any new information which may be targeted for reprocessing and continue to reprocess the existing targets. In this way, the therapist is regularly checking in with you about whether the treatment is working effectively and updating their plan accordingly.

What does it feel like to have EMDR therapy?

I asked Make Birth Better member Angie to describe her experience of EMDR following a traumatic birth. This is an extract from her blog for the Make Birth Better website:

'So what is EMDR therapy? The idea as it was explained to me is that when you have post-traumatic stress, the traumatic memories are stuck in the 'present' part of your brain and not filed away in the 'past' like other memories are. The therapy aims to get you to reprocess the memories so they can be properly filed. This is done by revisiting the traumatic memories while generating a 'rhythmic stimulus'. In my case, this was eye movements from side to side following my therapist's fingers, but I understand that tapping is also used.

What I really liked about the therapy was that, after the initial consultation, I didn't have to go over everything out loud in great detail or feel the need to articulate it in any particular way. During the EMDR itself, I needed only to think about a particular memory and let my mind go where it wanted. It would start off hard and uncomfortable with the memory seeming so very clear. Then as the eye movements continued, I'd progress through the memory, and by the end of that round

I would usually start to feel lighter and the memory would start to soften around the edges. I wasn't hypnotised; I was in control the whole time and could stop whenever I wanted to. Sometimes I cried. Sometimes I had physical sensations that went along with the memories.

Although it went well, I did find it to be incredibly draining. I would have my sessions in the morning and would be completely wiped out for the rest of the day, so I scheduled it for a day my son was at nursery. Emotions were all stirred up and sometimes I was actually thinking about the trauma more. I was warned about this, though, and I understood that it was the memories being reprocessed.

The other things I learned from my sessions were grounding techniques, which are strategies you can use to bring yourself into the present when the trauma feels too real. At the end of each session, or during if it was particularly hard, we would practice these. My therapist liked to throw a soft ball back and forth while going through an alphabetical list, such as naming a country (X is always really hard!). I've continued to use grounding outside therapy, too, when triggers come. My husband and I have sat in many NHS waiting rooms naming capital cities! I have also started practising yoga more regularly, which I find really helps me.

I finished my therapy right before Christmas last year after 12 sessions. My scores on the assessment for PTSD went down and I definitely felt better, though it took some time for things to settle down. And now after six months, although it's something that will always be a part of me and my story, I feel that my trauma has so much less impact on my day-to-day life.'

Here is Rochelle's experience of EMDR on the NHS:

'I was two years post the birth of my daughter, who was critically ill at birth and spent four weeks in intensive care in

four hospitals, and even had a flight in an RAF helicopter. I spent the first year of her life attributing my low mood and super high anxiety to the fact that I was tired. I realised when I went back to work that actually I couldn't continue how I was, so was lucky enough to have a referral straight to a women's health counsellor, who after the first visit or so suggested we try EMDR. I was apprehensive: I didn't feel I needed it, after all my daughter had survived, so I should just be getting on with it, surely?

The first few sessions were really tough, in the sense that I had so many "parts" as I call them, blocking the way to access my true thoughts. I had voices telling me I was silly, that I didn't need to talk about that memory or to tell me not to cry! So we took a break for a few weeks to work on addressing those "parts" and that really helped. It took some time, but eventually I was more able to access memories that I had burrowed away. Sometimes I would remember random memories like what I had for lunch on a particular day, certain conversations that I had, and also some of the more traumatic memories. I found it tiring; often I would need to pick my daughter up afterwards, which was exhausting as I would get headaches regularly afterwards. Where I could, I would try and take some time to myself when I got home to just allow my mind to stop. I found I sometimes had vivid dreams too.

I had the EMDR light bar therapy, with a green light, and preferred a specific speed of the light moving from side to side – my therapist was very careful to ensure that I was comfortable, and these little things made a big difference.

Overall, I believe the EMDR, coupled with talking therapy, pretty much turned my life around. There is no doubt that it takes courage to do EMDR therapy as you expose your thoughts in a way that can make you feel quite "naked".

However, I was lucky enough to have an amazing therapist, and I can also say now that I had great strength in facing my fears head on.'

An EMDR exercise

One of the key elements of EMDR is ensuring that you can reach a feeling of safety quickly. This ensures that you can stay calm and relaxed throughout the 'reprocessing' phases. One way of doing this is to create a safe place. When done with a therapist, they would use additional techniques to help really instill this 'safe place'. You can practice this visualisation every day:

- Picture a place that brings you feelings of calm and safety. This might be a real place or somewhere you imagine.
- Thinking of this place, how do you feel? What sensations can you feel in your body? What feelings does it raise for you?
- Can you hear anything? You might want to use soothing music or sounds to really enhance this feeling of relaxation.
- What would you call this safe place? Think of a word that you can use to describe it.

Practice bringing this word to mind and using it to visualise the safe place, and all of the feelings and physical sensations associated with it.

Perinatal distress

It may be that you are reading this book because you had a difficult birth, but there are other issues which are affecting you day to day at the moment. Perhaps you have been diagnosed with postnatal depression, but feel that you also have some symptoms of trauma due to your birth. Or that there are other factors which you have been thinking about more since you became a parent.

If you do have some symptoms of trauma, it's always useful to have them treated first as this can have positive impacts on other symptoms such as low mood and anxiety. However, there is a lot of overlap between different mental health conditions in this period – for example, we know that antenatal anxiety might make us more susceptible to developing postnatal depression. There are often common themes which emerge in research around perinatal mental health problems, such as loneliness, loss of autonomy, change in appearance, sexuality and limited social support. Some clinicians have suggested that rather than focussing on particular diagnoses, we should be moving towards a more holistic model of 'perinatal distress'.

We also know from a vast history of research that parental mental health difficulties can impact upon the relationship you develop with your baby. Approaches that allow you to bring your baby to sessions and work with the two (or more) of you together can really help to protect and enhance your relationship. These approaches can range from baby massage and positive parenting group sessions, to formal parent-infant psychotherapy.

With this in mind, you might want to seek a broader therapeutic approach once you feel your trauma has been resolved, or is only one part of a more complex difficulty. Many clinical psychologists who have specialist training in perinatal mental health will integrate different approaches in order to address the various different factors that could be impacting on you. You might be able to access this support through a talking therapies service, but more often this will involve a referral to a specialist perinatal mental health service, a parent-infant psychology service or similar, or seeking help from an independent practitioner.

Although within the NHS and the NICE guidance the focus is often on brief interventions such as CBT, the recent development of perinatal competencies and training by the Tavistock and Portman NHS Trust and Health Education England do emphasise the importance of more psychodynamic approaches and theories such as attachment theory and the importance of other significant and historical relationships. Some brief psychodynamic therapies are available on the NHS, such as Interpersonal Therapy and Dynamic Interpersonal Therapy, and longer term Psychodynamic Psychotherapy can also be beneficial.

Other treatments

Being Heard

After all of that description about somewhat complicated psychological interventions, one of the things which many people find, which isn't evidence-based but felt in our very bones, is that being *heard* is the most transformative experience of all. This may not be the case for those who might meet a PTSD diagnosis, where such retelling of a story could feel re-traumatising, but certainly it can be helpful for the majority of people who feel that certain aspects of their birth were difficult.

Sometimes we have this experience when we speak to a friend about our birth experience, or we seek help from a doula when planning a future birth, or when we see a kind healthcare professional who happens to ask about our experience of birth. But having someone listen is not the same as feeling heard.

Active listening is a counselling technique in which the listener isn't just passively taking in information, but puts aside their own judgements and preconceptions to fully engage with what they are hearing and also seeing in your behaviour and body language. They may then reflect back what they have heard. This can help you feel very understood, and can have a profound impact, particularly if you have felt ashamed about your birth experience.

Deep listening is a similar technique based in mindfulness, in which the listener actively engages with what is being said but hears it and reflects it back from a place of deep kindness and compassion:

> *'We spend most of our moments when someone is speaking, planning what we're going to say, evaluating it, trying to come up with our presentation of our self, or controlling the situation. Pure listening is a letting go of control. It's not easy and takes training...*
>
> *The bottom line is when we are listened to, we feel connected. When we're not listened to, we feel separate.'* Tara Brach, *The Sacred Art of Listening*

Of course, you can't find a 'listener' listed on any websites, but many different professionals are trained in these approaches: healthcare professionals such as midwives, health visitors and counsellors, and also mindfulness teachers, doulas and many others.

Debriefing

Most maternity services in the UK offer sessions variously known as 'birth reflections', 'birth debrief' and 'birth afterthoughts'. These are often held by a senior midwife, and frequently in the same location in which the birth took place.

Debriefing has been fairly controversial, and has been adopted in maternity services throughout the UK despite a lack of evidence to support its routine use – and there is some evidence that it could actually be re-traumatising. Where maternity notes are looked at in detail and more of an 'active listening' approach is used, it seems that this can be helpful rather than a more formal debriefing approach.

Many parents do find that these sessions help them to gain an understanding of what happened and why. Although they may not reduce psychological symptoms, anecdotally they are seen to be helpful for parents to feel they have 'aired their grievances', and that their experience has been validated, and for staff to reflect on their practice. It is recognised, though, that there is a need for a more standardised approach to these sessions and that they should not be used in place of a formal complaints procedure or to prevent litigation.

Peer and social support

For many women and birthing people, peer support and support from those around them can sometimes be the most healing thing of all. Trauma can leave us lacking in trust for others. In addition, all the messages after a traumatic birth that we 'should be grateful', leaving us questioning whether or not our feelings are valid, can add to feelings of shame. Speaking to others who have been through similar, and building up close relationships, can help us begin to feel a sense of trust again and normalise our feelings. It can also give us the impetus we need to seek further support.

The one disadvantage of more formal peer support, particularly in group form, is that it can be easy to end up in a room of people reliving their traumatic stories, which can not only trigger your own trauma memories, but can also lead to feelings of shame if you feel that others have 'had it worse'.

Here in the UK, the Birth Trauma Association has a peer support group on Facebook and is currently organising a peer support service via email. Kim Thomas, CEO of the Birth Trauma Association, told me about their peer support group:

'Our birth trauma support group on Facebook was formed in 2008, and now has more than 7,000 members, which probably

gives some idea of the scale of the need. The group, which is private, is exclusively for peer support – we only allow women who have experienced a traumatic birth, or their partners, to join.

Because it isn't always easy to gain access to professional help, the group provides a valuable lifeline for a lot of women. One of the pieces of advice often given to people with mental health problems is that they should talk – but that's only useful if you have someone who can listen. Many women tell us that friends, family and health professionals often dismiss their feelings of anger, grief and anxiety after a traumatic birth, telling them that they should "move on", or be grateful for the fact they have a healthy baby. Our Facebook group is a place where women know their story will be heard by people who understand what they're going through and won't judge them. It also enables women to ask for, and receive, advice and support on how to cope with triggers such as the baby's birthday or a close friend's pregnancy, or on topics such as making a complaint to the hospital.

We know women find the group useful because there's a constant flow of posts throughout the day, but some women also make a point of telling us how grateful they are. Some of them have even said that the group helped save their life, which is a wonderful testimony to the power of peer support, but also a terrible indictment of the lack of alternative support available to women experiencing postnatal PTSD.'

Although not specifically related to birth trauma, AIMS also has a helpline staffed by peer volunteers. They often help women and families think about the advocacy they might need, and will signpost to other services where appropriate. Debbie Chippington Derrick, Chair of AIMS, told me:

'AIMS supports all maternity service users to navigate the

system as it exists, and campaigns for a system which truly meets the needs of all. The AIMS Helpline volunteers are all experienced in providing information and support on pregnancy and birth issues. We do not give medical advice, but instead we focus on helping those who contact the Helpline to find the information that they need to make informed decisions which are right for them, and support them to have their decision respected by their healthcare providers. They are also able to provide a listening ear and practical support for women who are unhappy with their experiences.'

Finally, in the UK, Birthrights also has a helpline and can offer advice about your rights during pregnancy and childbirth.

In Australia, Debby Gould and Melissa Bruijn have run free 'Healing from Birth' meetings as part of their Birthtalk support and education organisation. They say:

'One of the most important initial steps on the healing journey from a bad birth can be the validation that comes from hearing other women's stories, and often hearing them express similar emotions and responses to those that you are experiencing.' (*How to Heal a Bad Birth*, p17)

Group therapy
Group therapy can offer psychoeducation about the symptoms of trauma as well as providing peer support and all of the benefits of this. While there are no specific studies currently available for group therapy for parents who have had a traumatic birth, studies in others who have traumatic symptoms have found group therapy can help to reduce those symptoms. Increasingly groups are being offered in talking therapies services, as they offer the opportunity to rapidly reach many people.

Jan Smith, a counselling psychologist in Huddersfield, runs

a group programme for parents following a traumatic birth. I asked her to tell me about how the group works:

'Our "Healing After Birth" intervention is a 12-week Acceptance and Commitment Therapy (ACT) group for mums experiencing a birth trauma. ACT is an evidence-based action-oriented approach to psychotherapy that stems from traditional behaviour therapy and CBT. Each session runs for two hours across 12 weeks, exploring a different birth trauma-related topic each week. The first hour focuses on the ACT intervention and the latter half is a support group. Examples of topics include "Psychoeducation of Trauma", "Writing Your Birth Story", "Accepting Difficult Thoughts", and "Healing Relationships" (with self and others). A number of perinatal mental health teams are hoping to run the group in 2019, and we aim to formally evaluate the efficacy of the group then. Anecdotally, women have found the group format has "normalised" their birth experience, and they've found it helpful to recognise their thoughts and not react to these.'

When group therapy is effective, it is often based on a particular psychological model such as group CBT. This enables tools and techniques to be taught, and also discourages the 'storytelling' that can be unhelpful in a less focused group.

Somatic techniques

The lifelong work of clinicians such as Bessel van der Kolk and Babette Rothschild has emphasised how much trauma can be held in the body, and highlighted how any techniques which can help to regulate the arousal system in the body (that powerful amygdala I keep mentioning!) will lead to enhanced feelings of safety.

As Bessel van der Kolk says:

'Mainstream Western psychiatric and psychological healing

traditions have paid scant attention to self-management. In contrast to the Western reliance on drugs and verbal therapies, other traditions from around the world rely on mindfulness, movement, rhythms and action. Yoga in India, tai chi and qigong in China, and rhythmical drumming throughout Africa are just a few examples… These techniques all involve physical movement, breathing and meditation.' (*The Body Keeps the Score*, p208).

Such techniques might include mindfulness, which allows us to attend to the shifts and changes in the body, rhythmic movement (such as dance or yoga) or sound (such as drumming), touch (such as bodywork therapy) or active experiences (such as self-defence classes).

Two such techniques have been growing in popularity recently.

Yoga
Yoga integrates both breath and bodywork, helping us to switch on the parasympathetic nervous system and switch off that threat response. There are a number of courses springing up for therapists and healthcare professionals to use yoga for trauma and other mental health conditions.

I asked Shweta Panchal, of the Minded Institute, to tell me about how yoga can be helpful after a traumatic birth. Shweta, a yoga and mindfulness therapist for mental health, told me that yoga can help us to work towards feeling safe through relaxation, teaches how to regulate our nervous system responses through breath work, improves interoception ('looking inside') and self-awareness and helps us to foster better communication.

There is growing evidence that yoga can have beneficial results for those with traumatic symptoms, at the very least as an adjunct to other treatments. For those who would prefer not to revisit traumatic memories in particular, it could be a very helpful support. Shweta said:

> *'Yoga can help to legitimize the experience of a traumatic birth by honouring and creating space for the somatic mind-body experience. Through breath, sound and mindful movement the story of the body can be told, expressed and eventually healed.'*

Closing the Bones
I feel as though a Closing the Bones ceremony should be offered to every new parent after giving birth. This postnatal massage, focused on the hips, is a deeply nurturing experience focused entirely on the mother's journey through pregnancy and birth. Originating from Ecuador, the stomach and hip area are massaged with warm oil, and rebozo (large shawls) are used to wrap and rock.

Although not a treatment for trauma, feeling held and comforted in this way can be a deeply powerful experience – if done with a trusted practitioner, this can speak to the physical symptoms of trauma, letting the body know that you are safe and held.

I asked Skevi Nicodemou, women's wellness therapist, how Closing the Bones can be beneficial for people after a difficult birth, and this is what she had to say:

> *'There is something deeply relaxing about being gently rocked, massaged and swaddled with love! In pregnancy and birth, everything opens up, physically and emotionally. The origin of Closing the Bones has deep roots in honouring the transition made into Motherhood, and closing a chapter of what was, and what wasn't – so it can be a great support and healing after birth. It's also "mothering the mother" which is often lacking.'*

Medication

The first-line treatment for PTSD should always be psychological therapy. However, for those people who don't wish to go through this process, are being held on a waiting list or would like some support in managing the symptoms of trauma, medication can be extremely beneficial.

If you feel that this would be helpful, please speak to a healthcare professional such as your GP or a psychiatrist.

Healing from physical trauma

Many women who have had a physical injury following childbirth find that it is difficult to find the right support for their recovery. 85% of women sustain some perineal tearing during birth (with 2.9% of those women having a third- or fourth-degree tear with some damage to the anal sphincter too). Half of women have a vaginal prolapse after birth, and nearly half suffer from urinary incontinence, yet few women are referred for specialist treatment.

In comparison to France, where postnatal women are automatically referred for gynaecological assessment and then a process of physical rehabilitation (called '*reéducation*'), in the UK women are offered very little follow up postnatally and are lucky if they are handed a leaflet on pelvic floor exercises.

If you are struggling after a physical injury, do speak to your GP or another healthcare professional. You may also wish to ask for a referral to a women's health physiotherapist.

Have a look at the Pelvic Roar campaign, and if you have had a third- or fourth-degree tear you can find support via Mothers with 4th Degree Tears and the MASIC Foundation, a charity that aims to reduce the incidence of birth injury.

Making a change

Many of the stories that we hear through Make Birth Better are stories of both trauma and negligence. Sometimes, sadly, birth trauma is caused by poor care. On many occasions trauma is caused by overstretched services, in which staff, despite the best of intentions, simply cannot offer the support they need to. On some occasions, trauma is caused by physical violation.

Making a complaint
Once you have recovered from some of the symptoms of trauma, you might wish to make a formal complaint about the treatment you received.

Initially, you can contact the service you were seen in – or you can ask someone to do this on your behalf. You can also speak to PALS, your local Clinical Commissioning Group (CCG), NHS England or the Care Quality Commission (CQC). There is information on the Make Birth Better website if you would like to find out more.

AIMS and Birthrights also have a lot of guidance on their websites to help you make a complaint.

If you feel that you have experienced unsafe practice, you can also contact the Healthcare Safety Investigation Branch (HSIB), a new independent organisation. As many healthcare professionals have described feeling unable to speak out about mistakes or working practices because of the culture of blame in many services, HSIB has been set up specifically not to attribute blame, but to conduct thorough investigations. This ensures that the emphasis is placed on reducing risks in the future. While not every report will be investigated, they are all logged and may be used in future investigations.

Sometimes the care you have received means that you might wish to take legal action against the professionals or Trust involved in your care. I asked Suzanne Munroe, a clinical negligence solicitor, to tell me a little about the process of seeking legal help:

'Having a baby is supposed to be a magical time but it doesn't always work out that way for many women. During pregnancy we look forward to meeting our baby, we learn all there is to know about how to have the "best birth" and how to "get it right". When something then goes wrong during the birth itself, which then may have a dramatic effect on the experience and may, in some cases, mean a mother cannot even look after her new baby, it is difficult to know where to turn. It might be some while afterwards that a mother (or someone in her family) realises that there could potentially be a legal case to investigate.

When clients do approach our firm, I always ask how we can help them to find answers, heal and move on with their lives. A lot of our clients have not only suffered physical injuries, but also psychological injuries, and I believe it is our job as lawyers to make sure our clients have the best outcome possible, whatever the conclusion of their legal case. We also have a responsibility to make sure that we don't make things worse by taking someone through the legal process without caring for them properly during it.

Our team of clinical negligence lawyers specialises in birth injury claims and has a wealth of experience in dealing with the difficult and sensitive issues that surround physical injury claims following birth. Young women can find themselves suffering distressing and embarrassing symptoms from physical birth injury – things they don't want to tell their doctor about or even sometimes their partner. Our job is to make sure we find out what has gone wrong and to see what we can do to try and improve women's lives by bringing a legal claim where we can.

There is a time limit for when you can bring a claim, but these time limits depend on the circumstances of the injury, when it occurred, whether the claim is for the mother, father or baby and many other factors. I would advise anyone considering contacting a lawyer not to let concerns about time limits stop you from seeking advice. If a claim is successful, any compensation can be life-changing for the family and help fund rehabilitation and support to help them move forward with their lives, and it is important to me that families do not miss out on compensation they deserve.

Often people prefer to approach a local lawyer about a potential claim, so they can see them in person at their offices and have someone they believe is easily accessible. Make sure that lawyer is an expert in these cases. I would recommend approaching someone who is a real specialist in clinical negligence claims.

Clinical negligence claims are usually very complicated and you need a specialist to really know the law and get the very best outcome for you. It also should be someone you feel comfortable with and can trust. I would like to think that my team take the time to get to know our clients, to ensure that they feel comfortable enough to trust us with their sensitive personal information, which we can then use properly to fight for the very best result, given each client's circumstances. I am passionate about making sure that we push for proper support and rehabilitation for all clients – it is not just about the amount of compensation, rather what difference that money makes for our clients.'

Creating change

Many people find that it can feel enormously healing to get involved in campaigns and advocacy following their own experience of trauma. At Make Birth Better, we hear from many parents who have used their own experience to influence practice in their local Trusts, to speak about their experiences at conferences or training days to inform professionals, or even to influence policy at governmental level.

You are welcome to come and join us at Make Birth Better if you would like to be involved in making a change. You may also wish to become involved with organisations such as the Birth Trauma Association, Birthrights and AIMS.

As part of the Maternity Transformation Programme, every local area also has a Maternity Voices Partnership meeting regularly and they are often looking for volunteers.

Emma Jane Sasuru is a mum of two who works with women following birth trauma. Following her own traumatic experience, she trained as a mindfulness and CBT practitioner. She also campaigns for maternity and perinatal mental health improvement, and is a lived experience expert who often speaks at conferences and events about her own experience. Emma told me:

'For me birth trauma was like a darkness that permeated every aspect of my life. I felt cocooned, unable to understand the many emotions that I struggled with daily. Fear, guilt, grief all became my companions. There were days where healing seemed to be impossible. It was lonely, I felt like no one really understood. My healing began when I finally felt heard, in the arms of women who listened to my story. We can never underestimate how powerful it is to have our experiences truly listened to and validated. Providing a safe space for those affected by birth trauma is so important; too often though we fail to do this. This is why I set up Unfold your Wings to offer those who felt alone like me hope. That they can believe it is possible to break free from the dark cocoon of birth trauma, spread their wings and find the light. I also believe that it is important that we look at prevention of birth trauma. This has moved me to use my lived experience to influence locally and nationally the care, services and policies in place to care for women and their families. This means I now work in the NHS supporting families, giving them the care that I know would have made such a difference to me. Sometimes bad things happen to us, but we can turn those experiences into opportunities to help others, change and improve things and give

a voice to those that need help and support. Yes, even trauma can lead us to something good: it provides us with a chance to make a difference and in turn helps heal ourselves.'

After a traumatic birth, you may feel that you will never recover. That the experience will always be there, affecting your memories of meeting your child and colouring those early days and months of parenthood with sadness.

I hope this chapter has demonstrated that not only can you recover from a difficult birth experience, but there are also many different ways to do so. You can think about what will work for you, and ask for what you are entitled to. There may be many different options which will work for you at different times. Dr Rebecca Moore, my Make Birth Better co-founder and a perinatal psychiatrist who takes a holistic approach to trauma recovery, says:

'Treatment for trauma needs to be holistic and developed collaboratively with each woman to provide a unique mix of care. This might include dietary change, blood testing, exercise planning, supplementation, therapy, medication, physiotherapy, social prescribing such as peer groups or networks, spiritual support or specialist psychosexual work. So one woman might opt for medication, couples therapy and a regular yoga practice. Another might want to use magnesium supplements, meditation, a peer group online and trauma focused CBT. Our treatment of trauma should be as subjective as a woman's response to trauma in the first place. We all deserve bespoke care.'

There is a growing area of research which explores 'post-traumatic growth'. For some, their traumatic experience can give them a sense of strength or purpose, or increased resilience. It's not easy, taking that first step towards recovery, but it can be a journey with a happy ending.

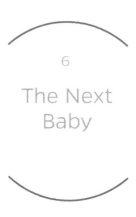

6

The Next Baby

Even considering another birth may feel impossible after a difficult first birth. Many women fear becoming pregnant again, and may also avoid sex, which of course makes becoming pregnant more difficult! Many couples make the decision not to have another child, or delay having another. Some researchers have suggested that the concern about having another child can actually feel like a threat, to the extent that this can trigger symptoms of trauma. Often it is not until we become pregnant, and experience the anxiety that this raises, that we realise how affected we were by our first birth.

However, birth after trauma can be incredibly healing with the right support. Beck and Watson (2010) suggested that the majority of women can go on to have a very healing birth after a traumatic first birth. Many of the women who take part in the Make Birth Better campaign describe positive subsequent birth experiences, whether that is vaginal birth or an elective C-section.

What seems to link these positive experiences is the amount

of support parents receive after a traumatic birth. Many parents find that second time around they have learned such a lot from their first experience – the things they definitely don't want to happen again, and the things they would really like to happen – and galvanise all the support they can.

If you are thinking of planning a birth after trauma, now is a great time to seek some help for any symptoms of trauma you are still experiencing. Change can happen very quickly in therapy when you are pregnant – not least because both you and the therapist are highly motivated!

Hearing stories

Often hearing others' birth stories can be the most reassuring aspect of preparing for a subsequent birth. Just as hearing of others' trauma can be normalising, hearing of others' positive experiences can give us the courage we really need at such an anxious time. Here I have chosen two very different second birth stories:

A healing VBAC, by Emma

'After my last birth – a planned home birth, which ended in an emergency C-section due to 'failure to progress', I was really clear that I wanted to try for a VBAC this time around. While I don't think my experiences affected my relationship with my first child, if anything it made them feel all the more precious, it definitely affected my relationship with myself, and my body, and health services. I felt flawed, a failure, and very angry that I didn't receive the support that I felt would have made that birth a positive experience.

So, this time around, as soon as I found out I was pregnant I hired a doula and started researching VBAC stats. I hadn't considered that I might plan a home birth again as I assumed it would be too risky, but at my booking-in appointment my midwife was encouraging. I then spoke to a doula, who was an enormous source of confidence for me throughout the pregnancy, and was there to answer all my anxious questions when I was full of doubt in my ability to give birth naturally. I also read tons of VBAC birth stories, all of the most positive being home births. I bought the Natal Hypnotherapy VBAC preparation CD, and listened to it as often as possible. And I joined a VBAC support group on Facebook, a group of ladies who were there day or night to offer words of encouragement. This made me start to think a home birth might be a good option for me, particularly as I was so scared of the pressure for intervention I had felt in hospital last time. After lots of discussion with my husband, the Supervisor of Midwives at our local hospital, and our doula, I decided to write a birth plan for each eventuality. My biggest fear was going into hospital too early and then being 'timed out', so the Supervisor of Midwives agreed we could book a home birth and be assessed at home before making a decision about whether or not to transfer to hospital. The community midwife who came to give me the home birth kit was very enthusiastic about my prospects and that spurred me on even more, when she left saying 'You're going to do this! You're going to have a great birth'. I was outwardly saying that my plan was to transfer to hospital if we had time, but my hope was that things would happen so quickly that we would choose to continue at home.

There were moments of course when I really questioned what I was doing, the risk of rupture (which although tiny could be catastrophic), whether it would just be easier to plan a C-section and not go through the uncertainty. But I really wanted to give myself a chance to give birth vaginally.

In the end I gave birth at home (in the bathroom!) with the support of my partner, two amazing midwives and my *wonderful doula.*

What really helped was ignoring the initial signs of labour, using a lot of relaxation techniques (I listened to my hypnobirthing track with the same oil burning each time so during labour, that smell really helped me stay relaxed), having reassurance from all of the people with me (I needed a lot of support, and they often said to me 'you're doing great' which spurred me on) and very discreet interventions from the midwives, checking the baby's heartrate, encouraging me to change position and asking about any pain.

When my son was born, he was so calm, no crying, just a few gulps and he slowly opened his eyes. It turned out he was in a similar position to his sister – her position was what I was told had caused her to 'get stuck' the first time. But with the right support, I was able to birth him. I had very minor tears and, just over a week later, felt almost back to normal. The best thing was sitting on my own sofa afterwards when everyone had gone, holding my baby, as compos mentis as I could be after that, not drug-addled and feeling invaded, just feeling like me.

I'm pleased to have had both experiences. Birth is hard bloody work and I feel less cheated about my first birth now I know what it entails. But more than ever I really understand the importance of the right support with experienced midwives in the right environment. Those midwives trusted my body as much as I did. This baby was the same size as my first, and in the same position, but they had faith that I could get him out on my own, they knew how to help me do it, they told me repeatedly that I could, and they trusted me enough not to intervene. I don't feel proud of myself, or empowered or any of those things I felt cheated of last time. More than anything, I feel vindicated. I knew I could do it, and now I have.'

A healing C-section birth, by Vikki

'I am nine-months post an amazing elective C-section experience for my second child after a traumatic birth with my first three years prior (a massive post-partum haemorrhage and intensive care stay).

The whole C-section experience was calm, positive and felt far more 'natural' than my vaginal birth. Post-delivery my daughter was in my arms within four minutes (wrapped up) and we were having skin-to-skin in theatre within 10 minutes. I was breastfeeding in recovery after 45 minutes and on the ward after two hours. It was wonderful and very healing after my first birth.

What really helped me was having open and honest conversations with consultants. I was vocal about what I wanted. I met with the anaesthetist the day before to talk through exactly what would happen and cover any remaining questions. I had lots of plans in place to let me take it easy in recovery, although my recovery was far better this time than with my first birth! I could walk to the corner shop by day four!

I also took all the medication I was offered to keep any pain down. I used medication that was safe for use during breastfeeding, and it meant I could get up and about a little, which helped my recovery.'

A second trauma

Sometimes, of course, a second birth is not the healing experience that you have been longing for. You may be reading this book having had not one, but more traumatic experiences. Here, Vicki talks about how she recovered from two traumatic births:

'When I think of my two births, I view them very differently, but no less traumatic. My first was physically traumatic where

I suffered a haemorrhage and my son was taken away to the NICU. My second birth was spontaneous at home, where I gave birth very quickly. Because they were both so different it took me a long time to recognize my second birth was traumatic too. Just because there wasn't a big physical event and my new baby didn't go into NICU it didn't mean that giving birth on my own, with no guidance at home in less than an hour, was any less traumatic. It took going to therapy for postnatal depression and the therapist asking me if I was okay about the birth for me to realise I wasn't. She sympathised, she asked me questions and unlocked how I really felt. No one had asked that before. But once I did recognize them both equally and began to verbalise my birth trauma, I began to move on from the trauma. I sought comfort from the support I received from others who had been through similar things, after I shared publicly on social media. The flashbacks are less frequent and I feel I can talk about them in a more positive way.'

If you have experienced a subsequent trauma, please do look at Chapter 5 on healing and the 'Seeking Help' section at the back.

Birth planning

Many women who have had difficult or traumatic births feel understandably angry that the plans they had carefully formulated went out of the window, and often express a sense that they were 'set up to fail' as they hadn't been aware of potential negative outcomes. Both lead us to question the usefulness of birth planning, and even whether it could be harmful.

The temptation is to say that birth planning is a bit pointless. Why plan something that is unlikely to go your way? So then we soften our requests. We refer to them as birth 'preferences' instead of plans, we ensure that the language on the plan remains flexible and polite instead of appearing demanding, and we go into birth believing that our plans are nothing more than a fairytale.

But actually, birth planning is an essential component of pregnancy and antenatal care. For those giving birth, it gives us the opportunity to do our research, to talk to people and find out about others' experiences, to hear about different outcomes and consider what we might choose in different eventualities. As birth partners, it gives us the chance to hear about how we can best support our partner and ensure that specific anxieties or concerns are aired before the birth. As healthcare professionals, it is a quick and easy way to hear what is important to the families we are working with, and a starting point for discussion.

We know that going into birth with positive expectations also increases your likelihood of a satisfactory experience. So why are we dissuaded from making plans, and finding out information with which to create those expectations?

In any other circumstance in our lives that had the power to change our future – such as a wedding, a job interview or a house move – we would spend many hours planning and doing our research (even knowing that these too are circumstances during which things may happen outside of our control). When we've experienced that plan going completely awry, it can be tempting not to make another. And when we know how stretched maternity services are, again it might feel that we're just setting ourselves up to 'fail' again. But we don't need to chuck the birth plan out with the bathwater! It just means we need to include that situation in our planning. If you're not likely to have a midwife you know during your birth, perhaps you'd like to think about an additional birth partner or a doula? If you know the services near you are struggling, can you have a conversation with your midwife about how you can still get what you need from them? If you are one of a queue of women waiting to see a stressed-out midwife, might there be an opportunity to speak again on the phone if you have questions left unanswered?

What is a useful plan?

The type of birth plan we're talking about matters. Many birth plans only cover an ideal scenario. This can reflect the belief that if we don't enter into birth positively, the anxiety raised by negative thoughts could interfere with oxytocin and make it more likely we'll have a difficult birth. But let's think about that for a moment. What raises anxiety in your day-to-day life? If you were going to a new place and felt nervous about how you would get there, would you ignore your worry and set off on your journey without a map? Or would you do a bit of research, think about the different ways of arriving and plan your journey? Might you also get advice from people who make that journey often, or who have made the journey before?

When we go into any new situation, or a situation full of uncertainty, we have a choice. We can deny, or we can plan. We know from previous chapters that denial doesn't remove those symptoms of trauma. Pulling them out and looking at them is what makes them less frightening. It can help to think through not only an ideal Plan A, but also Plan B, C and D – including a worst-case scenario allowing all of your fears to be aired. It means that, even if everything goes completely off piste, you can still feel you have exercised choice and control over what is happening, and those around you know what you need from them in order to offer the best support they can.

There's also the dilemma of how to plan, but you can really draw from your previous experiences here. What do you wish you'd known then? Who do you wish had been around? What do you wish they'd done? Your maternity notes will have a section to offer guidance on the kind of topics you can start to think about, and there are lots of example birth plans online. Milli Hill's book *The Positive Birth Book* has a very comprehensive section on birth planning, including icons you can use to create a visual birth plan (to ensure the key elements of your plan are easy to see).

One of the big questions many people are left with is whether to plan for a physiological birth or whether to choose an elective C-section. You are entitled (thanks to the NICE guidelines) to request a C-section if this is your preference. Discussing your options, and the risks and benefits of different interventions (and non-interventions too), can often be the most helpful part of the birth planning process. Don't forget that as well as asking for things, you also have a right to decline them.

Some parents also worry about whether a birth plan has the potential to cause conflict with healthcare professionals. Especially if you found a healthcare professional was not receptive to your plan first time around, it might feel like too much to go through that process again. But in many ways, our caution over birth planning – essentially making it clear what we want – is reminiscent of the deferential attitudes towards medics that are dying out. We still consider this when writing birth plans, making sure that our language is polite and unchallenging. Of course we don't want to challenge those who are tasked to care for us during birth, but equally we don't need to feel that we have to be careful about their feelings being hurt. In my eyes, birth should be a collaboration between all of the parties involved. In this way, there is a trust that a woman or birthing person will do what is best for them and their baby… and that a healthcare professional will also do what is best for them.

So birth planning can be a crucial part of pregnancy, helping you think about your hopes and fears and providing a starting point for collaboration with those around you.

A birth squad

You may also want to put together a 'team' of people around you who can offer you support, advice and reassurance. There is now a 'Tokophobia Toolkit' available to guide clinicians in working with women who are experiencing fear around birth, which you can access yourself on the internet and show to your midwife or consultant. This suggests a recommended timeline for the different care options you should be offered (such as early appointments with a consultant, referrals to psychological therapies and continuity of carer).

Midwife

Following a traumatic birth, you may be entitled to work with a specialist mental health midwife. They can offer you support around any distress you might be experiencing, help you access additional support if necessary and also plan this birth in collaboration with you.

Louise Nunn is a specialist mental health midwife in London and was involved in developing a pathway for women with tokophobia. She told me:

'The most important reason that I got involved in this area of care is that sometimes the focus ends up being purely on the decision whether to "allow" a woman to give birth by caesarean, but that's only one part of the issue. Actually what women want to have is a positive birth experience – regardless of the actual way they give birth. The primary aim is not to coerce women into giving birth vaginally (although the results show that the majority do end up having successful and very positive vaginal births), but that they feel supported, and decisions are made in partnership.'

Obstetrician

You might also be offered consultant-led care. They will be

able to discuss different birth options with you. Caroline Wright outlined to me the support that obstetricians aim to give families:

> 'I want mothers, partners and families to know that obstetricians and midwives are working towards the same goal as mums – which is always getting mum and baby safely through labour and delivery, but also respecting birth plans/ wishes. We are often mothers ourselves, and we are on your side! I think obstetricians are often sold as the bad guys, but all they want is good outcomes for mums and babies. I hope that we are able to put our experience and knowledge across to mums in the right way to help them when decisions feel difficult.
>
> We know these are special moments in your life and we strive to get it right! And I really hope that for the most part, we do. We all know the pressures on the NHS and staffing problems can make our job more difficult, but we are constantly trying to improve and deliver first-class maternity care, because that is what women and families deserve. This is what we would want for ourselves, our families, our friends and our colleagues. We will keep listening, keep working, keep changing until we get it right.'

Doula

Many women, birthing people and their partners find having a doula can be tremendously reassuring. They can offer you, and your partner, support, reassurance and advocacy. They also ensure that you have some continuity of care, and they know you and your birth plan well so they can make your wishes known during labour. Although doulas can seem an expensive investment, many doulas offer payment plans and reduced rates.

I asked Natalie Meddings, doula and founder of Tell Me a

Good Birth Story and author of *Why Home Birth Matters*, how she supports women and birthing people after a traumatic first birth:

> *'An essential role for me, as a doula, is to revisit the first birth and untangle the events around it. Sometimes this can bring a sigh of relief, if by talking the mother comes to see that her birth was disturbed by the circumstances around her or that the obstetric care she received was essential. It can also help us think about how she was treated and how this can be different next time around. Once we start to prepare for the next birth, a doula can help to form a personal plan and to protect the mother's space and advocate for her throughout her birth. This extra support can really help birth be simple and straightforward second time around.'*

Independent midwife

Although this can seem like a prohibitively expensive option for many people, independent midwives can often offer the continuity of care, individualised support, time and patience that can be difficult to find within the NHS. If this is an option that appeals to you, do discuss options with your local independent midwives, as many also offer payment plans.

Liz Nightingale, a retired independent midwife, told me:

> *'Fundamentally, independent midwives offer their clients time – which helps a truly trusting and mutually respectful relationship. We care about our clients. They care about us. This mutuality grows through continuity of carer. And this means that even, or perhaps especially, those who are survivors of previous trauma find the way we work so beneficial and helpful.'*

Peer support

There are many peer support groups on social media. As well as the Birth Trauma Association support group and the Make Birth Better pages, there are also support groups such as 'VBAC Support', 'Beyond Birth Trauma' and many other local groups.

Natalie Meddings has also set up the Tell Me a Good Birth story website, which provides a 'birth buddy' for people looking for reassurance and support from those who have been through similar experiences.

While the Positive Birth Movement was not created specifically for those who have experienced a traumatic birth, many use these groups to gain information and peer support while planning a subsequent birth. Milli Hill, founder of the PBM, said:

> '...some women attend our groups after a traumatic birth first time round, when preparing for their second baby – a time that can be filled with anxiety for many women who know they don't want a "repeat experience". Our groups are not set up to help women process their trauma, however the groups can still be helpful in providing a place for women to think differently about their next birth. They can hear positive birth stories, find out more about their rights and choices in the birth room, and this feeling of knowing that they have lots of options and that what happens to them is their choice, can be very reassuring.'

Planning a second baby after a traumatic experience can feel like a huge mountain to climb, but most people do go on to have a positive subsequent birth. Many women describe their second birth as completing their recovery from their difficult birth. Jo Page, Make Birth Better contributor, talks about her second birth as being a transformative experience, not healing the trauma but giving her a new perspective:

> '...*within minutes he was out and peeping over the screen at me, my beautiful baby, the one I never dreamt I'd be brave enough to have, the one that gave me the true feelings of the special moments after giving birth... so anyone planning this after a trauma, it was the best thing that could have happened to me.*'

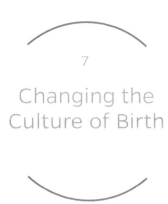

7

Changing the
Culture of Birth

'If women are in a perinatal environment where there is positive emotion, optimism, social support, where women actively cope, feel mastery and have a sense of purpose or meaning, they will flourish.' (Ayers, 2017)

What makes birth trauma so unique among traumatic experiences is that there are such clear ways to prevent or reduce its impact, if we look only at the care people are offered. Having heard these same stories over the past 10 years, it raises questions for me about why we as a society are accepting how frequently women come out of birth feeling bruised. It's not that birth can be difficult – because we know that people can come out of objectively traumatic experiences without symptoms of PTSD or trauma. In my mind, it's that we are sending many people into maternity systems which are traumatising. This, perhaps, is indicative of how little we value our women, parents and children.

The whole maternity journey gives us a unique opportunity to reach people that we often miss. The clear fact is that, often, we are getting it wrong. 81% of women surveyed by the Royal College of Obstetricians and Gynaecologists in 2017 had experienced some form of mental health difficulty in the perinatal period, yet only 1 in 5 of them had been referred for support. While 1 in 25 experience PTSD after birth, at least a third of women report some symptoms of trauma. We know that half of women who have perinatal mental health difficulties will not try to seek help. This is despite how frequently we are in contact with health services before, during and after birth. For people who are living with multiple difficulties and may usually avoid contact with services, this period of time is a particular chance to offer support. As family members and friends, we tend to avoid conversations about birth, and buy into the dichotomies around 'good' and 'bad' births.

Why don't women, birthing people and their partners feel confident confiding in us, as healthcare professionals, as friends, as partners? If we can ensure that parents are properly supported prior to, during and after birth, we can change things not just for parents, but their children too.

For this to still be happening, despite increased funding in maternity services and perinatal mental health, indicates that funding is not the problem (or, perhaps, not the only problem). We also need to look at cultures within maternity services – which stretch staff to the limit, and then blame them when things go wrong – and how we talk about birth as a society. At the very least, we need to consider how we can stop causing harm, and then think about how we can further prevent it.

Currently, this means thinking about how birth, preventing birth trauma and offering rapid and quality support to those who have experienced a traumatic birth is being implemented at a local level. National guidelines are one thing – but it is clear that at present these are often not being followed locally. Continuity of carer is one such example. There has been a huge amount of research highlighting the importance of continuous support during labour – making it more likely a person will have a shorter labour, less likely that they will have a c-section or instrumental birth, and more likely that they will be satisfied (Hodnett et al., 2011). Continuity of carer is one of the key recommendations from the *Better Births* report. Yet, as a recent AIMS statement points out, there is an urgent need to ensure that this recommendation is delivered in realistic and sustainable ways across the country.

There has been a move throughout trauma-*focused* research and practice to think about trauma-*informed* ways of working, so that we are not just looking at individuals, but creating whole systems which acknowledge how trauma can impact on individuals and groups. This moves us away from identifying who is traumatised, and towards policies, protocols and interventions which actively avoid re-traumatising for all involved and support people in their ability to cope. In maternity, for example, this might be as simple as avoiding internal examinations to assess progress. Antenatally, there would be a need to ensure that information is shared so that fully informed consent can be gained for interventions (or the choice not to intervene) and women, birthing people and their partners feel a sense of control and agency over their choices (and their bodies). But, more widely, there is a need to ensure that everyone within a service (staff as well as patients) is treated with compassion and respect. This might involve clearer communication between professionals, examining cultures where bullying and fear are common.

In early 2019 we developed a conceptual model to help professionals and parents think about how we can use some of the ideas and issues raised in this book in order to prevent birth trauma and reduce its impact on everyone. This model was created in collaboration with the parents and professionals involved in the Make Birth Better network, and you can learn more about it on our website (see 'Model').

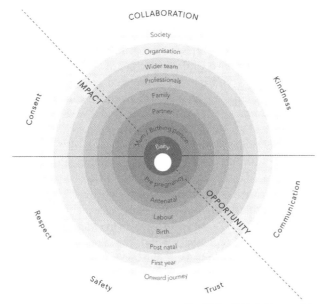

COLLABORATION

Society

Organisation

Wider team

Professionals

Family

Partner

Mum / Birthing person

Baby

Pre pregnancy

Antenatal

Labour

Birth

Post natal

First year

Onward journey

IMPACT

OPPORTUNITY

Consent

Kindness

Respect

Communication

Safety

Trust

The Make Birth Better model

We are beginning to provide resources, training, consultation and supervision for healthcare and birth professionals, and our training manual highlights the many examples of best practice in trauma-informed birth and maternity care. We believe small changes could make a huge difference. Just by taking on the core values outlined around the edges of the model, we believe we could see a reduction in traumatic birth experiences. In addition, learning particular skills for use during the maternity journey could have a great impact at many different points of opportunity. For example, midwives, obstetricians or anaesthetists who can spot signs of dissociation during labour and use gentle grounding techniques could reduce symptoms of PTSD after birth. Susan Ayers has suggested that, as the meanings attributed to events are so influential in PTSD, if professionals sensitively discussed different possible outcomes before and during labour and birth, women might be less likely to make negative appraisals. If we then quickly and kindly approached families with risk factors for birth trauma after the birth, we could intervene early and ensure that women and their families are not left living with the consequences of a difficult birth.

There are also exciting innovations in this field. In Blackpool, expert in trauma-informed care Mickey Sperlich has been working with BetterStart to develop trauma-informed and trauma-specific interventions in the perinatal period. In Warwick, Kirstie McKenzie-McHarg, a clinical psychologist working within a maternity service, and her team have developed a simple 'pink sticker' system to highlight the women and families who might need additional support. This, alongside whole-team training in perinatal mental health and birth trauma has seen a 44% drop in women being referred to the psychology service due to birth trauma. In Switzerland, the simple introduction of a computer game (such as Tetris) for women immediately following an emergency C-section birth reduced the number of intrusive memories a week later (Horsch et al., 2017).

There is a groundswell, driven not only by national and international policy guidelines, but by birth activists and women and families, saying '#TimesUp'. But to ensure these changes happen, we need to find out what is happening in our local services and encourage our local commissioners. We need to keep talking, keep informing and keep supporting one another.

Where women, partners and staff are supported, birth can be a transformative experience. If we can get this right, we can prevent the spread of trauma through future generations. We can set people up well for their parenting journey. We can turn the birth story into a positive one. Imagine how powerful that would be.

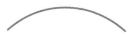

Seeking Help

If you would like support, please speak first to your GP or another healthcare professional to find out what is in your local area.

Have a look at the Make Birth Better website. There are lots of resources on there as well as a map of services offering support after a difficult birth.

Please ensure that, when seeking support, your practitioner has the appropriate qualifications to work with trauma, is registered with a professional body and has suitable supervision in place.

If you feel that you are in a crisis and cannot cope with your current feelings, please seek an urgent appointment with your GP or visit A&E. Please don't forget that there is always hope and that people can and do recover from mental health difficulties.

Useful Websites

Make Birth Better *www.makebirthbetter.org*
Birthrights *www.birthrights.org.uk*
Birth Trauma Association *www.birthtraumaassociation.org.uk*
AIMS *www.aims.org.uk*
Unfold Your Wings *www.unfoldyourwings.co.uk*
Andrew Mayers *www.andrewmayers.info*
Fathers Reaching Out *www.reachingoutpmh.co.uk*

For General Mental Health Support

MIND *www.mind.org.uk* Infoline 0300 123 3393
Samaritans *www.samaritans.org* Helpline 24/7 call 116 123

For Help With Relationships and Sex

Tavistock Relationships *www.tavistockrelationships.org*
Relate *www.relate.org.uk*
The Havelock Clinic *www.thehavelockclinic.com*

For Help Bonding with your Baby

Parent Infant Partnership UK *www.pipuk.org.uk*
Association for Infant Mental Health *www.aimh.org.uk*

For Help With Birth Injury

MASIC Foundation (for Mothers with Anal Sphincter Injuries)
     masic.org.uk
Mothers with 4th Degree Tears *motherswith4thdegreetears.
     wordpress.com*
Pelvic Roar *www.pelvicroar.org*

For Help after a Birth Related Incident

The Healthcare Safety Investigation Bureau offers independent
     investigations and also has a comprehensive list of resources
     *www.hsib.org.uk/public-patients/support-advice-patients-carers-
     families*

For Help after a NICU experience

Bliss *www.bliss.org.uk*
Support for NICU Parents *www.support4nicuparents.org*

For Help After the Death of a Baby

SANDS *www.sands.org.uk*
Tommy's *www.tommys.org*

References

Introduction: It's Not Just About a Healthy Baby

Hill, M. (2017). *The Positive Birth Book: A new approach to pregnancy, birth and the early weeks*. London: Pinter & Martin Limited.

Meddings, N. (2017). *How to have a Baby: Mother-gathered guidance on birth and new babies*. London: Eynham Press.

Mental Health Taskforce. (2016). *The five year forward view for mental health*. United Kingdom: Mental Health Taskforce.

NHS Improving Quality. (2015). *Improving access to perinatal mental health services in England – A review*. United Kingdom: NHS Improving Quality.

NHS. (2016). *Maternity transformation programme*. Retrieved March 18, 2019, from https://www.england.nhs.uk/mat-transformation/

World Health Organization. (2018). *WHO recommendations: intrapartum care for a positive childbirth experience*. Geneva: World Health Organization.

Chapter 1: What is Trauma?

American Psychiatric Association. (2013). *Diagnostic and statistical manual of mental disorders* (5th ed.). Washington, DC: American Psychiatric Association.

Brewin, C. R. (2015). Re-experiencing traumatic events in PTSD: new avenues in research on intrusive memories and flashbacks. *European Journal of Psychotraumatology, 6*(1), 27180. doi: 10.3402/ejpt.v6.27180

Brewin, C. R., Dalgleish, T., & Joseph, S. (1996). A dual representation theory of posttraumatic stress disorder. *Psychological Review, 103*(4), 670-686. doi: 10.1037/0033-295X.103.4.670

Brewin, C. R., Lanius, R. A., Novac, A., Schnyder, U., & Galea, S. (2009). Reformulating PTSD for *DSM-V*: Life after criterion A. *Journal of Traumatic Stress, 22*(5), 366–373. doi: 10.1002/jts.20443

van der Kolk, B. (2014). *The body keeps the score: Mind, brain and body in the transformation of trauma*. London: Penguin Random House.

Weathers, F. W., & Keane, T. M. (2007). The criterion A problem revisited: controversies and challenges in defining and measuring psychological trauma. *Journal of Traumatic Stress, 20*(2), 107-121. doi: 10.1002/jts.20210

World Health Organization. (2018). *International statistical classification of diseases and related health problems* (11th ed.). Retrieved from https://icd.who.int/browse11/l-m/en

Chapter 2: Birth Trauma: A Silent Epidemic

Abelsohn, K. A., Epstein, R., & Ross, L. E. (2013). Celebrating the "other" parent: Mental health and wellness of expecting lesbian, bisexual, and queer non-birth parents. *Journal of Gay & Lesbian Mental Health, 17*(4), 387-405. doi: 10.1080/19359705.2013.771808

American Society of Anesthesiologists. (2018). *Postpartum depression linked to mother's pain after childbirth: New study underscores importance of managing pain during recovery*. Retrieved March 18, 2019, from www.sciencedaily.com/releases/2018/10/181014142700.htm

Andrews, E.E. (2011) Pregnancy with a physical disability: One psychologist's journey. *Spotlight on Disability Newsletter*, American Psychological Association

Ayers, S. (2004). Delivery as a traumatic event: Prevalence, risk factors, and treatment for postnatal posttraumatic stress disorder. *Clinical Obstetrics and Gynecology, 47*(3), 552-567. doi: 10.1097/01.grf.0000129919.00756.9c

Ayers, S., Bond, R., Bertullies, S., & Wijma, K. (2016). The aetiology of post-traumatic stress following childbirth: a meta-analysis and theoretical framework. *Psychological Medicine, 46*(6), 1121-1134. doi: 10.1017/S0033291715002706

Ayers, S., Wright, D. B., & Thornton, A. (2018). Developmental of a measure of postpartum PTSD: The city birth trauma scale. *Frontiers in Psychiatry, 9*(409). doi: 10.3389/fpsyt.2018.00409

Basu, M., Smith, D., & Edwards, R. (2016). Can the incidence of obstetric anal sphincter injury be reduced? The STOMP experience. *European Journal of Obstetrics & Gynecology and Reproductive Biology, 202*, 55-59. doi: 10.1016/j.ejogrb.2016.04.033

Beck, C. T. (2006). The anniversary of birth trauma: failure to rescue. *Nursing Research, 55*(6), 381-390. Retrieved from https://journals.lww.com/nursingresearchonline/Abstract/2006/11000/The_Anniversary_of_Birth_Trauma__Failure_to_Rescue.2.aspx

Beck, C. T., Driscoll, J. W., & Watson, S. (2013). *Traumatic childbirth.* Abingdon: Routledge.

Birth Trauma Association. (n.d.). *Post natal post traumatic stress disorder.* Retrieved March 18, 2019, from http://www.birthtraumaassociation.org.uk/publications/Post_Natal_PTSD.pdf

Bliss for Babies Born Premature or Sick. (2018). *Bliss calls for better psychological support on neonatal units.* Retrieved March 18, 2019, from https://www.bliss.org.uk/news/2018/bliss-call-for-better-psychological-support-on-neonatal-units

Cardwell, V. & Wainwright, L. (2018), *Making Better Births a reality for women with multiple disadvantages: A qualitative peer research study exploring perinatal women's experiences of care and services in north-east London* . Retrieved March 2019 from https://www.birthcompanions.org.uk/media/Public/Resources/Ourpublications/RDA_BC-REPORT_WEB_FINAL.pdf

Crawley, R., Lomax, S., & Ayers, S. (2013). Recovering from stillbirth: the effects of making and sharing memories on maternal mental health. *Journal of Reproductive and Infant Psychology, 31*(2), 195-207. doi: 10.1080/02646838.2013.795216

Draper, E. S., Gallimore, I. D., Kurinczuk, J. J., Smith., P. W., Boby, T., Smith, L. K., & Manktelow, B. N. (2018). *MMBRACE-UK perinatal mortality surveillance report: UK perinatal deaths for births from January to December 2016.* Leicester: The Infant Mortality and Morbidity Studies, Department of Health Sciences, University of Leicester.

Dunn, A. B., Paul, S., Ware, L. Z., & Corwin, E. J. (2016). Perineal injury during childbirth increases risk of postpartum depressive symptoms and inflammatory markers. *Journal of Midwifery & Women's Health, 60*(4), 428-436. doi: 10.1111/jmwh.12294

Fassler, J. (2015). *How doctors take women's pain less seriously.* Retrieved March 18, 2019, from https://www.theatlantic.com/health/archive/2015/10/emergency-room-wait-times-sexism/410515/

Hayes, A. (2018). *Postnatal pain and the link with postnatal depression.* Retrieved March 18, 2019, from https://motherswellnesstoolkit.wordpress.com/2018/12/08/postnatal-pain-and-the-link-with-postnatal-depression/

Hodnett, E. D., Gates, S., Hofmeyr, G. J., Sakala, C., & Weston, J. (2011). Continuous support for women during childbirth. *Cochrane Database Systematic Reveiw, 16* (2),

Hoffman, K. M., Trawalter, S., Axt, J. R., & Oliver, M. N. (2016). Racial bias in pain assessment and treatment recommendations, and false beliefs about biological differences between blacks and whites. *Proceedings of the National Academy of Sciences of the United States of America, 113*(16), 4296-4301. doi: 10.1073/pnas.1516047113

Horsch, A., & Ayers, S. (2016). Chapter 39 – Childbirth and stress. In G. Fink (Ed.), *Stress: Concepts, cognition, emotion, and behaviour* (pp. 325-330). London: Elsevier Inc.

Iles, J., & Pote, H. (2015). Postnatal posttraumatic stress: A grounded theory model of first-time mothers' experiences. *Journal of Reproductive and Infant Psychology, 33*(3), 238-255. doi: 10.1080/02646838.2015.1030732

Kiesel, L. (2017). *Women and pain: disparities in experience and treatment.* Retrieved March 18, 2019, from www.health.harvard.edu/blog/women-and-pain-disparities-in-experience-and-treatment-2017100912562

Lee, D.A.. (2005). The perfect nurturer: A model to develop a compassionate mind within the context of cognitive therapy. *Compassion: Conceptualisations, Research and use in Psychotherapy*. 326-351.

Malouf R., McLeish J., Ryan S., (2017) 'We both just wanted to be normal parents': a qualitative study of the experience of maternity care for women with learning disability. *BMJ Open* 2017;7

McKenzie-McHarg, K., Ayers, S., Ford, E., Horsch, A., Jomeen, J., Sawyer, A., . . . Slade, P. (2015). Post-traumatic stress disorder following childbirth: an update of current issues and recommendations for future research. *Journal of Reproductive and Infant Psychology, 33*(3), 219-237. doi: 10.1080/02646838.2015.1031646

McLeish, J., & Redshaw, M. (in press). Maternity experiences of mothers with multiple disadvantages in England: A qualitative study. *Women and Birth.* doi: 10.1016/j.wombi.2018.05.009

Munafó, M. R., Nosek, B. A., Bishop, D. V. M., Button, K. S., Chambers, C. D., du Sert, N. P., . . . Ioannidis, J. P. A. (2017). A manifesto for reproducible science. *Nature Human Behaviour, 1*(0021). doi: 10.1038/s41562-016-0021

National Institute for Health and Care Excellence (April 2018). *Antenatal and postnatal mental health: clinical management and service guidance, Clinical guideline [CG192].* Retrieved March 2019 https://www.nice.org.uk/guidance/CG192

NHS, *NHS Maternity Statistics, 2016-2017* (Nov 2017). Retrieved March 2019 from https://digital.nhs.uk/data-and-information/publications/statistical/nhs-maternity-statistics/2016-17

Royal College of Obstetricians and Gynaecologists (2018). *OASI Care Bundle.* Information retrieved March 2019 from https://www.rcog.org.uk/OASICareBundle

Seng, J., & Taylor, J. (2015). *Trauma informed care in the perinatal period.* London: Dunedin Academic Press Limited.

Singhal, A., Tien, Y.-Y., & Hsia, R. Y. (2016). Racial-ethnic disparities in opioid prescriptions at emergency department visits for conditions commonly associated with prescription drug abuse. *PLOS ONE, 11*(8), e0159224. doi: 10.1371/journal.pone.0159224

Sperlich, M. (2015). How does focusing on posttraumatic stress disorder shift perinatal mental health paradigms?. In J. Seng & J. Taylor (Eds.), *Trauma informed care in the perinatal period* (p. 42-56). Edinburgh: Dunedin Academic Press.

The Royal College of Midwives. (2016). *Interventions in normal labour and birth.* London: Royal College of Midwives.

Walker, K. (2017). What issues do lesbian co-mothers face in their transition to parenthood? *Perspective, 34*. Retrieved from https://www.nct.org.uk/sites/default/files/related_documents/Walker%20K%20What%20issues%20do%20lesbian%20co-mothers%20face%20in%20their%20transition%20to%20parenthood.pdf

Walker, S., van Rijn, B. B., Macklon, N. S., & Howe, D. T. (2014). PLD.31 The rising rate of labour induction: what is causing the trend? *Archives of Disease in Childhood – Fetal and Neonatal Edition, 99*(1), A115. doi: 10.1136/archdischild-2014-306576.331

Weisse, C. S., Sorum, P. C., Sanders, K. N., & Syat, B. L. (2001). Do gender and race affect decisions about pain management?. *Journal of General Internal Medicine, 16*(4), 211-217. doi: 10.1046/j.1525-1497.2001.016004211.x

Chapter 3: Experiencing Birth Trauma

Astrup, J. (2018). *More midwives needed for 'better births'*. Retrieved March 18, 2019, from https://www.rcm.org.uk/news-views-and-analysis/news/more-midwives-needed-for-better-births

Bohren, M. A., Vogel, J. P., Hunter, E. C., Lutsiv O, Makh, S. K., Souza, J. P., . . . Gülmezoglu, A. M. (2015). The mistreatment of women during childbirth in health facilities globally: A mixed-methods systematic review. *PLOS Medicine, 12*(6), e01001847. doi: 10.1371/journal. pmed.1001847

Bryanton, J., Gagnon, A. J., Hatem, M., & Johnston C. (2008). Predictors of early parenting self-efficacy: Results of a prospective cohort study. *Nursing Research 57*(4), 252-259. doi: 10.1097/01.NNR.0000313490.56788.cd

Button, S., Thornton, A., Lee, S., Shakespeare, J., & Ayers, S. (2017). Seeking help for perinatal psychological distress: a meta-synthesis of women's experiences. *British Journal of General Practice, 67*(663), 692-699. doi: 10.3399/bjgp17X692549

Dahlberg, U., & Aune, I. (2013). The woman's birth experience – the effect of interpersonal relationships and continuity of care. *Midwifery, 29*(4), 407-415. doi: 10.1016/j.midw.2012.09.006

Elmir, R., Schmied, V., Wilkes, L., & Jackon, D. (2010). Women's perceptions and experiences of a traumatic birth: a meta-ethnography. *Journal of Advanced Nursing, 66*(10), 2142-2153. doi: 10.1111/j.1365-2648.2010.05391.x

Garthus-Niegel, S., Ayers, S., van Soest, T., Torgersen, L. & Eberhard-Gran, M. (2015). Maintaining factors of posttraumatic stress symptoms following childbirth: A population-based, two-year follow-up study. *Journal of Affective Disorders, 172,* 146-152. doi: 10.1016/j.jad.2014.10.003

Gottvall, Karin & Waldenström, Ulla. (2002). Does a Traumatic Birth Experience Have an Impact on Future Reproduction?. *BJOG : an international journal of obstetrics and gynaecology.* 109. 254-60.

Iles, J. & Pote, H. (2015). Postnatal posttraumatic stress: A grounded theory model of first-time mothers' experiences. *Journal of Reproductive and Infant Psychology, 33*(3), 238-255. doi: 10.1080/02646838.2015.1030732

Lokugamage, A. U., & Pathberiya, S. D. C. (2017). Human rights in childbirth, narratives and restorative justice: a review. *Reproductive Health, 14*(17), 1-8. doi: 10.1186/s12978-016-0264-3

Mobbs, N., Williams, C., & Weeks, A. D. (2018). *Humanising birth: Does the language we use matter?*. Retrieved from https://blogs.bmj.com/bmj/2018/02/08/humanising-birth-does-the-language-we-use-matter/

Moore, D., Drey, N., & Ayers, S. (2017). Use of online forums for perinatal mental illness, stigma and disclosure: An exploratory model. *Journal of Medical Internet Research Mental Health, 4*(1), e6. doi: 10.2196/mental.5926

NCT. (2017). *Hidden Half Campaign*. Retrieved March 18, 2019, from https://www.nct.

org.uk/get-involved/campaigns/hidden-half

Newton, N., & Newton, M. (1962). Mothers' reactions to their newborn babies. *JAMA, 181*(3), 206-210. doi: 10.1001/jama.1962.03050290028005

Pickles, C. (2017). *Reflections on obstetric violence and the law: What remains to be done for women's rights in childbirth?*. Retrieved March 18, 2019, from https://www.law.ox.ac.uk/research-and-subject-groups/international-womens-day/blog/2017/03/reflections-obstetric-violence-and

Prevatt, B-S., & Desmarais, S. L. (2018). Facilitators and barriers to disclosure of postpartum mood disorder symptoms to a healthcare provider. *Maternal and Child Health Journal, 22*(1), 120-129. doi: 10.1007/s10995-017-2361-5

Reed, R., Sharman, R., & Inglis, C. (2017). Women's descriptions of childbirth trauma relating to care provider actions and interactions. *BMC Pregnancy and Childbirth, 17*(21). doi: 10.1186/s12884-016-1197-0

Royal College of Obstetricians and Gynaecologists (2017). *O&G Workforce Report 2017.* London: Royal College of Obstetricians & Gynaecologists.

Ryding, E. L., Wijma, K., & Wijma, B. (1998). Experiencing emergency cesarean section: A phenomenological study of 53 women. *Birth, 25*(4), 246-251. doi: 10.1046/j.1523-536X.1998.00246.x

Chapter 4: The Second Victim

Areias, M. E., Kumar, R., Barros, H., & Figueiredo, E. (1996). Correlates of postnatal depression in mothers and fathers. *The British Journal of Psychiatry, 169*(1), 36-41. doi: 10.1192/bjp.169.1.36

Ayers, S., Eagle, A., & Waring, H. (2006). The effects of childbirth-related post-traumatic stress disorder on women and their relationships: A qualitative study. *Psychology, Health & Medicine, 11*(4), 389-398. doi: 10.1080/13548500600708409

Beck, C. T., Driscoll, J. W., & Watson, S. (2013). *Traumatic childbirth.* Abingdon: Routledge.

Beck, C.T.& Gable, R.K. (2012). A Mixed Methods Study of Secondary Traumatic Stress in Labor and Delivery Nurses. *Journal of obstetric, gynecologic and neonatal nursing,* 41(6):747-60

Chan, K. L., & Paterson-Brown, S. (2002). How do fathers feel after accompanying their partners in labour and delivery?. *Journal of Obstetrics and Gynaecology, 22* (1), 11-15. doi: 10.1080/01443610120101628

Delicate, A., Ayers, S., Easter, A., & McMullen, S. (2018). The impact of childbirth-related post-traumatic stress on a couple's relationship: a systematic review and meta-synthesis. *Journal of Reproductive and Infant Psychology, 36*(1), 102-115. doi: 10.1080/02646838.2017.1397270

Etheridge, J., & Slade, P. (2017). "Nothing's actually happened to me": the experiences of fathers who found childbirth traumatic. *BMC Pregnancy Childbirth, 17*(80). doi: 10.1186/s12884-017-1259-y

Hanson, S., Hunter, L. P., Bormann, J. R., & Sobo, E. J. (2009). Paternal fears of childbirth: A literature review. *Journal of Perinatal Education, 18*(4), 12-20. doi: 10.1624/105812409X474672

Harris, M. (2015). *Men, love & birth.* London: Pinter & Martin.

Hinton, L., Locock, L., & Knight, M. (2014). Partner experiences of "near-miss" events in pregnancy and childbirth in the UK: A qualitative study. *PLOS ONE, 9*(4), e91735. doi: 10.1371/journal.pone.0091735

Johnson, M. (2002). An exploration of men's experience and role of childbirth. *Journal of Men's Studies, 10*(2), 165–179.

Kainz, G., Eliasson, M., & von Post, I. (2010). The child's father, an important person for the mother's well-being during the childbirth: a hermeneutic study. *Health Care for Women International, 31*(7), 621-635. doi: 10.1080/07399331003725499

Leinweber, J., Creedy, D. K., Rowe, H., & Gamble, J. (2017) Responses to birth trauma and prevalence of posttraumatic stress among Australian midwives. *Women and Birth, 30*(1), 40-45. doi: 10.1016/j.wombi.2016.06.006

Matthey, S., Barnett, B., Kavanagh, D. J., & Howie, P. (2001). Validation of the Edinburgh postnatal depression scale for men, and comparison of item endorsement with their partners. *Journal of Affective Disorders, 64*(2-3), 175-184. doi: 10.1016/S0165-0327(00)00236-6

Olin, R., & Faxelid, E. (2003). Parents' needs to talk about their experiences of childbirth. *Scandinavian Journal of Caring Sciences, 17*(2), 153–159. doi: 10.1046/j.1471-6712.2003.00105.x

Pezaro, S., Clyne, W., Turner, A. P., Fulton, E. A., & Gerada, C. (2015). "Midwives Overboard!" Inside their hearts are breaking, their makeup may be flaking but their smile stays on. *Women and Birth, 29*(3), 59-66. doi: 10.1016/j.wombi.2015.10.006

Quillivan, R. R., Burlison, J. D., Browne, E. K., Scott, S. D., & Hoffman, J. M. (2016). Patient safety culture and the second victim phenomenon: Connecting culture to staff distress in nurses. *Joint Commission Journal on Quality and Patient Safety. 42*(8), 377-386. doi: 10.1016/S1553-7250(16)42053-2

Royal College of Midwives (2017) *Work, Health and Emotional Lives of Midwives in the United Kingdom: The UK WHELM study* . Retrieved March 2019 from https://www.rcm.org.uk/media/2924/work-health-and-emotional-lives-of-midwives-in-the-united-kingdom-the-uk-whelm-study.pdf

Royal College of Obstetricians and Gynaecologists (2018). *O&G Workforce Report* 2018. Retrieved March 2019 from https://www.rcog.org.uk/globalassets/documents/careers-and-training/workplace-and-workforce-issues/rcog-og-workforce-report-2018.pdf

Schumacher, M., Zubaran, C., & White, G. (2008). Bringing birth-related paternal depression to the fore. *Women & Birth, 21*(2), 65-70. doi: 10.1016/j.wombi.2008.03.008

Simpson, M., Schmied, V., Dickson, C., & Dahlen, H. G. (2018). Postnatal post-traumatic stress: An integrative review. *Women & Birth, 31*(5), 367-379. doi: 10.1016/j.wombi.2017.12.003

Thomas, K. (2013). *Birth Trauma: A guide for you, your friends and family to coping with post-traumatic stress disorder following birth.* Nell James Publishers

Ullstrom, S., Sachs, M. A., Hansson, J., Ovretveit, J., & Brommels, M. (2014). Suffering in silence: a qualitative study of second victims of adverse events. *BMJ Quality & Safety, 23*(4), 325-331. doi: 10.1136/bmjqs-2013-002035

Wahlberg, Å., Andreen Sachs, M., Johannesson, K., Hallberg, G., Jonsson, M., Skoog Svanberg, A., & Högberg, U. (2017). Post-traumatic stress symptoms in Swedish obstetricians and midwives after severe obstetric events: a cross-sectional retrospective survey. *BJOG: An International Journal of Obstetrics & Gynaecology, 124*(8), 1264-1271. doi: 10.1111/1471-0528.14259.

Waterman, A.D., Garbutt, J., Hazel, E., Dunagan, W. C., Levinson, W., Fraser, V. J., & Gallagher, T. H. (2007). The emotional impact of medical errors on practicing physicians in the United States and Canada. *Joint Commission Journal on Quality and Patient Safety, 33*(8), 467-476. doi: 10.1016/S1553-7250(07)33050-X

Webb, R., & Ayers, S. (2014). Cognitive biases in processing infant emotion by women with depression, anxiety and post-traumatic stress disorder in pregnancy or after birth: A systematic review. *Cognition and Emotion, 29*(7), 1278-1294. doi:

10.1080/02699931.2014.977849

West, C.P., Huschka, M. M., Novotny P. J., Sloan, J. A., Kolars, J. C., Habermann, T. M., & Shanafelt, T. D. (2006). Association of perceived medical errors with resident distress and empathy: a prospective longitudinal study. *JAMA, 296*(9), 1071-1078. doi: 10.1001/jama.296.9.1071

Wu, A. (2000). Medical errors: the second victim. *BMJ, 320*(726). doi: 10.1136/bmj.320.7237.726

Wyllie, C., Platt, S., Brownlie, J., Chandler, A., Connolly, S., Evans, R., Kennelly, B., . . . Scourfield, J. (2012). *Men, suicide and society: why disadvantaged men in mid-life die by suicide.* Surrey: Samaritans.

Chapter 5: Healing

Ayers, S., McKenzie-McHarg, K., & Eagle, A. (2007). Cognitive behaviour therapy for postnatal post-traumatic stress disorder: case studies. *Journal of Psychosomatic Obstetrics & Gynaecology, 28*(3), 177-184. doi: 10.1080/01674820601142957

Ayers, S., Wright, D. B., & Thornton, A. (2018). Development of a measure of postpartum PTSD: The City Birth trauma scale. *Frontiers in Psychiatry, 9*(409). doi: 10.3389/fpsyt.2018.00409

Baxter, J. (2017). *Listening to women after birth: their perceptions of postnatal support and the potential value of having a postnatal debriefing session with a midwife.* (Unpublished doctoral dissertation). City, University of London, London, United Kingdom.

British Psychological Society. (2018). *Survey of mental health workforce finds many services compromised by staff vacancies.* Retrieved March 22, 2019, from https://www.bps.org.uk/news-and-policy/survey-mental-health-workforce-finds-many-services-compromised-staff-vacancies

Garthus-Niegel, S., Ayers, S., van Soest, T., Torgersen, L. & Eberhard-Gran, M. (2015). Maintaining factors of posttraumatic stress symptoms following childbirth: A population-based, two-year follow-up study. *Journal of Affective Disorders, 172,* 146-152. doi: 10.1016/j.jad.2014.10.003

Horsch, A., & Ayers, S. (2016). Chapter 39 – Childbirth and stress. In G. Fink (Ed.), *Stress: Concepts, cognition, emotion, and behaviour* (pp. 325-330). London: Elsevier Inc.

Brujin, M., & Gould, D. (2016). *How to heal a bad birth: Making sense, making peace and moving on.* Birthtalk.org

Lapp, K., Agbokou, C., Peretti, C.-S., & Ferreri, F. (2010). Management of post traumatic stress disorder after childbirth: a review. *Journal of Psychosomatic Obstetrics & Gynecology, 31*(3), 113-122. doi: 10.3109/0167482X.2010.503330

McKenzie-McHarg, K. (2013). *Treatment of PTSD following childbirth: the importance of context.* Retrieved March 22, 2019, from https://blogs.city.ac.uk/birthptsd/2013/07/15/treatment-of-ptsd-following-childbirth-the-importance-of-context/

McKenzie-McHarg, K., Ayers, S., Ford, E., Horsch, A., Jomeen, J., Sawyer, A., . . . Slade, P. (2015). Post-traumatic stress disorder following childbirth: an update of current issues and recommendations for future research. *Journal of Reproductive and Infant Psychology, 33*(3), 219-237. doi: 10.1080/02646838.2015.1031646

Mind. (2013). *We still need to talk: A report on access to talking therapies.* London: Mind.

Mitchell, K. S., Dick, A. M., DiMartino, D. M., Smith, B. N., Niles, B., Koenen, K. C., & Street, A. (2014). A pilot study of a randomized controlled trial of yoga as an intervention for PTSD symptoms in women. *Journal of Traumatic Stress 27*(2), 121–128. doi: 10.1002/jts.21903

Muzik, M., Marcus, S. M., & Flynn, H. A. (2009). Psychotherapeutic treatment options for perinatal depression: emphasis on maternal-infant dyadic outcomes. *The Journal of Clinical Psychiatry*, 70(9), 1318-1319. doi: 10.4088/JCP.09com05451

Sandström, M., Wiberg, B., Wikman, M., Willman, A.-K., & Högberg, U. (2008). A pilot study of eye movement desensitisation and reprocessing treatment (EMDR) for post-traumatic stress after childbirth. *Midwifery*, 24(1), 62-73. doi: 10.1016/j.midw.2006.07.008

Schwartze, D., Barkowski, S., Strauss, B., Knaevelsrud, C., & Rosendahl, J. (2017). Efficacy of group psychotherapy for posttraumatic stress disorder: Systematic review and meta-analysis of randomized controlled trials. *Psychotherapy Research*, 27, 1-17. doi: 10.1080/10503307.2017.1405168.

Seidler, G., & Wagner, F. (2006). Comparing the efficacy of EMDR and trauma-focused cognitive-behavioral therapy in the treatment of PTSD: a meta-analytic study. *Psychological Medicine*, 36(11), 1515-1522. doi: 10.1017/S0033291706007963

Shapiro, F (2018). *Eye Movement Desensitization and Reprocessing (EMDR) Therapy, Third Edition: Basic Principles, Protocols, and Procedures*. Guilford Press

van der Kolk, B. (2014). *The body keeps the score: Mind, brain and body in the transformation of trauma*. London: Penguin Random House.

Chapter 6: The Next Baby
Beck, C. T., & Watson, S. (2010). Subsequent childbirth after a previous traumatic birth. *Nursing Research*, 59(4), 241-249. doi: 10.1097/NNR.0b013e3181e501fd

Chapter 7: Changing the Culture of Birth
Ayers, S., Bond, R., Bertullies, S., & Wijma, K. (2016). The aetiology of post-traumatic stress following childbirth: a meta-analysis and theoretical framework. *Psychological Medicine*, 46(6), 1121-1134. doi: 10.1017/S0033291715002706

Ayers, S., & Shakespeare, J. (2015). Should perinatal mental health be everyone's business?. *Primary Health Care Research & Development*, 16(4), 323-325. doi: 10.1017/S1463423615000298

BirthChoice. (2013). *Trends in freestanding midwife-led units in England and Wales*. London: Royal College of Midwives

Button, S., Thornton, A., Lee, S., Shakespeare, J., & Ayers, S. (2017). Seeking help for perinatal psychological distress: a meta-synthesis of women's experiences. *British Journal of General Practice*, 67(663), 692-699. doi: 10.3399/bjgp17X692549

Coates, R., Ayers, S & de Visser, R. (2014). Women's Experiences of postnatal distress: a qualitative study. *BMC Pregnancy & Childbirth*, 14(14), 359. doi: 10.1186/1471-2393-14-359.

Horsch, A., Vial, Y., Favrod, C., Harari, M. M., Blackwell, S. E., Watson, P., . . . Holmes, E. A. (2017). Reducing intrusive traumatic memories after emergency caesarean section: A proof-of-principle randomized controlled study. *Behaviour Research and Therapy*, 94, 36-47. doi: 10.1016/j.brat.2017.03.018

AIMS Call to Action https://www.aims.org.uk/journal/item/better-births-call-to-action

Olander, E. K., McKenzie-McHarg, K., Crockett, M., & Ayers, S. (2014). Think pink! A sticker alert system for psychological distress or vulnerability during pregnancy. *British Journal of Midwifery*, 22(8), 590-595. doi: 10.12968/bjom.2014.22.8.590

Moore, D., Drey, N., & Ayers, S. (2017). Use of online forums for perinatal mental illness, stigma and disclosure: An exploratory model. *Journal of Medical Internet Research Mental Health*, 4(1), e6. doi: 10.2196/mental.5926

Royal College of Obstetricians & Gynaecologists. (2017). *Maternal mental health – Women's voices*. London: Royal College of Obstetricians & Gynaecologists.

Index

abandoned, feeling 29, 52
Abuela Doulas 36
abuse in childhoods *see* history of abuse/trauma
Acceptance and Commitment Therapy (ACT) 115
active listening 110–11
active management of labour 41
acute stress reactions 18
Adverse Childhood Experiences (ACEs) 15
advocacy and campaigning work 121–3
afterthoughts sessions *see* debriefs/ reflections
AIMS (Association for Improvements in the Maternity Services) 113–14, 119, 122, 140
alcohol, as coping strategy 32
'all that matters is a healthy baby' 9–14, 60–1, 85, 113
amygdala 20, 88, 115–16
Andrews, Erin E. 38
anger 100–1
anniversaries 32, 76
antenatal education 56–8, 66, 67, 68, 70–1, 140
anxiety 18, 26, 28, 40, 56–7, 74, 109, 124
Areias, M. E. 67
arousal and reactivity 19, 21 *see also* hyperarousal/hypervigilance
Asian communities 36
assault 50
attachment/bonding 54–5, 68, 73, 74, 76, 109
Aune, I. 52
austerity cuts to the NHS 93
Australia 114
avoidance, as symptom 19, 24, 27, 28, 55, 59
Ayers, Susan 25, 27–8, 68, 74, 138, 141

baby
    death of 33–5, 50
    illness of 32–3
    trauma in the relationship with 73–6
'bad mother' narratives 43–5
Beck, Cheryl 25, 28, 32, 56, 77, 124
being heard 62, 64, 110–11, 122
bereavement care 34
Better Births 41–2, 140
BetterStart 142
Birth Companions 39
birth planning 129–37
Birth Reflections sessions 62
birth squads 133
birth stories
    being heard 110–11
    healthcare professionals' 81
    as part of healing treatments 91–2, 97, 98–9
    peer and social support 112
    Positive Birth Movement 57
    prevalence of negative 57
    as research source 46–7
    and societal trauma 65–6
    during subsequent pregnancies 125–8
birth trauma
    definition of 24–6
    diagnosis of 23, 25, 40
    experiences of 46–64
    misdiagnosed as postnatal depression 62
    statistics on 25, 139
Birth Trauma Association 30, 62, 112, 122, 136
Birth Trauma Awareness Week 46
birthdays, as triggers 32, 76
Birthrights 114, 119, 122
Birthtalk 114
Black and Minority Ethnic (BAME)

communities 31, 36
blame 19, 22, 44, 46, 59, 78
Bliss 32, 33
Body Keeps the Score, The (van der Kolk) 22
body scanning 104
bodywork therapy 116
Bohren, M. A. 50–1
bonding/attachment 54–5, 68, 73, 74, 76, 109
Brach, Tara 111
brain processing of trauma 20, 88
Braithwaite, Candice 36
breastfeeding 55, 75–6
breathing techniques 88–9, 102
Brewin, Chris 16, 20, 21
Broca's area 20
Bruijn, Melissa 114
Bryanton, J. 49
Button, S. 60

campaigning and advocacy work 121–3
Care Quality Commission 119
Cassidy, Tina 41
Centre for Maternal and Child Health Research at City University 27
Children's Services 61
Chippington Derrick, Debbie 113–14
City Birth Trauma Scale 27
Clark, David 21, 97
Clinical Commissioning Group 119
clinical negligence 119–21
closing the bones ceremonies 117
Cochrane reviews 43
coercion 50, 51, 52
coercive language 30, 49
Cognitive Behavioural Therapy (CBT) 21–2, 29, 63, 91, 94, 97–103
compassion 45, 78–9, 111, 140
compassionate care 40, 42
compassion-focused therapies 45
complaints, making 93, 101, 119–21

complex PTSD 22
complex trauma 39–40, 109
consent 40, 42, 50, 51, 140
continuity of care 42, 134, 139–40
control, sense of 28, 29, 49, 82, 140
coping strategies 28, 32
cortisol 20
C-section births 29, 53, 80, 82, 127, 132, 142

Dahlberg, U. 52
danger, sensing 21, 22
death of baby 33–5
debriefs/reflections 62, 91–2, 111–12
deep listening 111
definition of birth trauma 24–6
definition of trauma 15–22
delay in appearance of symptoms 54
depression 28, 40 *see also* postnatal depression
desensitisation 104
detachment 55
Diagnostic and Statistical Manual of Mental Disorders (DSM-V) 16, 19, 27
diatheses-stress model of birth trauma 27–8
disabilities, women with 36, 38–9
disconnection 71
dismissal of women's pain 30–1
dissociation 21, 28, 29, 55, 141
doctors 76–84, 134
doulas 63, 126, 134–5
Driscoll, J. W. 75
dual awareness 104
dual representation theory 20

early motherhood 53–6
Ehlers, Anke 21, 97
Elmir, R. 47
emergency C-sections 29
empathy 83
episodic memory 20

evidence-based treatments 91
expectations of birth 57, 130
Eye Movement Desensitisation and Reprocessing (EMDR) 91, 103–8

failure, birth experienced as 44, 59, 97, 99
fear 19, 25, 28, 29, 42, 49, 59
feminism 31
fight/flight/freeze 20, 88, 96
Five Year Forward Plan (NHS) 11, 94, 95
flashbacks 18, 24, 53, 73, 80, 99
'force bigger than me' 47–51

Gable, R. K. 77
Garthus-Niegel, S. 54
gender roles 67
Gottvall, K. 56
Gould, Debby 114
grief 33–5
grounded theory methodology 46–7
grounding 88–9, 98, 99, 102, 104–5, 106
group therapy 114–15
guilt 54, 55, 61 see also self-blame
Gurney, Karen 37, 72

Harris, Mark 68
Hayes, Anya 30
healing 56, 63, 81, 86–123
healthcare professionals
    and birth plans 132
    and the experience of birth trauma 51–3
    role of 41
    trauma in 76–84
Healthcare Safety Investigation Branch 119
heard, being 62, 64, 110–11, 122
hearing about a stressor event 16 see also witnessing
held, feeling 117

helplessness 19, 22, 29, 69, 99
helplines 113–14, 144
'Hidden Half' (NCT Campaign) 60
Hill, Milli 13, 57, 132, 136
hippocampus 20
history of abuse/trauma 15, 22, 28, 39–40, 92, 98–9, 102
history of mental health problems 28
Hodnett, E. D. 140
holistic care 122
home births 125–7
Horne, Hannah 81–3
Horsch, A. 142
hotspots 29, 97
How to Have a Baby (Meddings) 13
How to Heal a Bad Birth 62, 69, 114
hyperarousal/hypervigilance 26, 27, 53, 74, 83

iatrogenic harm 41
ignored, feeling 29
Iles, J. 56
ill babies 32–3
imagery 98
Impact of Events Scale 27
improvements to birth services 63–4, 138–42
Improving Access to Psychological Therapies (IAPT) programme 11, 93, 94, 95
incontinence 118
independent midwives 135
information during pregnancy 56–8 see also antenatal education
informed consent 40, 42, 50, 51, 140
insecure attachment 74
International Classification of Diseases (ICD-11) 17, 22
interpersonal factors 29
Interpersonal Therapy and Dynamic Interpersonal Therapy 110
interventions during birth 29, 41, 42, 51, 82, 140

Janet, Pierre 21
judgment, fearing others' 59
Jung, Carl 81

Kay, Adam 77–8
Keane, T. M. 17
kindness, treatment with 52, 111 *see also* compassion
Kitzinger, Sheila 41

learning disabilities, women with 38–9
Lee, D. A. 45
legal cases 119–20
LGBTI+ people 37–8, 67, 69–70
light bar therapy 107
listening to women 64, 110–11 *see also* being heard
lived experience experts 122
location of trauma, revisiting 91–2, 98, 111
Lokugamage, A. U. 50
long-term effects of birth trauma 13, 54
long-term therapies 110
Lord, Mars 36
low mood 19, 54, 89 *see also* postnatal depression

Make Birth Better 32, 39, 47, 48, 57, 62, 63–4, 84, 86, 119, 121, 140–1
Make Motherhood Diverse 36
Malouf, R. 38
MASIC 118
maternity services, as cause of trauma 41–2
Maternity Transformation Programme 11, 42, 95, 122
Maternity Voices Partnership 122
Matthey, S. 67
Mayers, Andy 13, 69
McKenzie-McHarg, Kirstie 97, 142
Meddings, Natalie 13, 134–5, 136
media portrayals of birth 57, 85
medicalisation of childbirth 41–2, 85

medication 118
memory
    becoming safe again 87–8, 89
    buried 107
    City Birth Trauma Scale 27
    flashbacks 18, 24, 53, 73, 80, 99
    fragmented 21
    integration 98, 100, 103–8
    making memories of a stillborn baby 33
    memory-focused treatments 87–9, 96, 97–103
    nightmares 21, 24, 53
    of previous abuse 28
    processing of trauma 18, 20–1
    unwanted memories 18
mental health *see also* perinatal mental health
    mental health services (NHS) 93–4
    partners' 62, 67–8
    stigma 60, 61–2
midwives
    bereavement specialists 33–4
    independent midwives 135
    more time to be with women 64
    positive relationships with mothers 52
    shortages of 52
    specialist midwives 12, 133
    during subsequent pregnancies 126, 133
    trauma in 76–84
migrant communities 36
MIND We still need to talk report 96
mindfulness 83, 111, 116, 117
minority communities 35–7
misdiagnosis 40
misinformation 57
missed diagnosis of birth trauma 40
missing out on early motherhood 54–5
MMBRACE report 36–7
Mobbs, N. 52
Moore, D. 61, 62